MRCP1
Pocket Book
2

Basic Sciences
Infectious Diseases
Neurology
Psychiatry

Third Edition

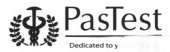

PasTest

Dedicated to y

MRCP1
Pocket Book
2

Basic Sciences
Infectious Diseases
Neurology
Psychiatry

Philip Ambery MRCP MFPM
Benjamin Clark MBChB MRCP DTM&H
Geraint Rees MB BCh PhD FRCP
Elizabeth Sampson MD MRCPsych

Third Edition

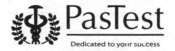

Dedicated to your success

© 2008 PASTEST LTD
Egerton Court, Parkgate Estate
Knutsford, Cheshire, WA16 8DX
Telephone: 01565 752000

Third edition 2008
Second edtion 2004
First edition 2002

ISBN: 1 905635 04 4
ISBN: 978 1 905635 047

A catalogue record for this book is available from the British Library.

The information contained within this book was obtained by the author from reliable sources. However, while every effort has been made to ensure its accuracy, no responsibility for loss, damage or injury occasioned to any person acting or refraining from action as a result of information contained herein can be accepted by the publishers or author.

Text prepared by Keytec Typesetting Ltd, Bridport, Dorset
Printed and bound in the UK by CPI Antony Rowe

CONTENTS

INTRODUCTION

PasTest's MRCP Part 1 Pocket Books are designed to help the busy examination candidate to make the most of every opportunity to revise. With this little book in your pocket, it is the work of a moment to open it, choose a question, decide upon your answers and then check the answer. Revising 'on the run' in this manner is both reassuring (if your answer is correct) and stimulating (if you find any gaps in your knowledge).

The MRCP Part 1 examination consists of two papers, each lasting three hours. Both papers contain 100 'Best of Five' questions (one answer is chosen from five options). Questions in each specialty are randomised across both papers. *No marks are deducted for a wrong answer.*

One-best-answer/'Best of Five' MCQs
An important characteristic of one-best-answer MCQs is that they can be designed to test application of knowledge and clinical problem-solving rather than just the recall of facts. This should change (for the better) the ways in which candidates prepare for MRCP Part 1.

Each one-best MCQ has a question stem, which usually contains clinical information, followed by five branches. All five branches are typically homologous (eg all diagnoses, all laboratory investigations, all antibiotics etc) and should be set out in a logical order (eg alphabetical). Candidates are asked to select the ONE branch that is the best answer to the question. A response is not required to the other four branches. The answer sheet is, therefore, slightly different from that used for true/false MCQs.

A good strategy that can be used with many well-written one-best MCQs is to try to reach the correct answer without first scrutinising the five options. If you can then find the answer you have reached in the option list, then you are probably correct.

One-best-answer MCQs are quicker to answer than multiple true/false MCQs because only one response is needed for each question. Even though the question stem for one-best-answer MCQs is usually longer than for true/false questions, and therefore takes a little longer to read carefully, it is reasonable to set more one-best than true/false MCQs for the same exam duration – in this instance 60 true/false and 100 one-best are used in exams of 2 hours' duration.

Application of Knowledge and Clinical Problem-Solving
Unlike true/false MCQs, which test mainly the recall of knowledge, one-best-answer questions test application and problem-solving. This makes them more effective test items and is one of the reasons why testing time can be reduced. In

order to answer these questions correctly, it is necessary to apply basic knowledge – not just the ability to remember it. Furthermore, candidates who cannot reach the correct answer by applying their knowledge are much less likely to be able to choose the right answer by guessing than they were with true/false MCQs. This gives a big advantage to the best candidates, who have good knowledge and can apply it in clinical situations.

Books like the ones in this series, which consist of 'Best of Five' questions in subject categories, can help you to focus on specific topics and to isolate your weaknesses. You should plan a revision timetable to help you spread your time evenly over the range of subjects likely to appear in the examination. PasTest's **Essential Revision Notes for MRCP** by P Kalra will provide you with essential notes on all aspects of the syllabus.

CONTRIBUTORS

THIRD EDITION

Basic Sciences
Philip Ambery MRCP MFPM, Honorary Clinical Fellow, Addenbrookes Hospital, Cambridge

Infectious Diseases
Philip Ambery MRCP MFPM, Honorary Clinical Fellow, Addenbrookes Hospital, Cambridge
Benjamin Clark MBChB MRCP DTM&H Specialist Registrar in Infectious diseases, Sheffield Teaching hospitals NHS Trust

Neurology
Professor Geraint Rees MB BCh PhD FRCP, University College London & National Hospital for Neurology & Neurosurgery, London

Psychiatry
Elizabeth Sampson MD MRCPsych, MRC Research Fellow, Department of Mental Health Sciences, Royal Free and University College Medical School, London

SECOND EDITION

Basic Sciences
Shani Esmail BSc MB Chir MRCP, Clinical Research Fellow in Clinical Pharmacology And Therapeutics, Western general Hospital, Edinburgh.
David W Ray PhD MRCP, Senior Lecturer in Medicine and Honorary Consultant in Endocrinology University of Manchester and Manchester Royal Infirmary, Manchester.
Edward Tobias BSc MBChB MRCP PhD, Glaxo-Wellcome Clinical Research Fellow And Honorary consultant in Medical Genetics Department of Medical Genetics University of Glasgow, Glasgow.

Infectious Diseases Infectious Diseases – Pocket Book 4
Ian Cropley MA MBBS MRCP Consultant in Infectious Diseases and HIV, Royal Free Hospital, London.
Alan J Hakim MA MRCP, Consultant Rheumatologist and General Physician, Whipp's Cross University Hospital, London, Honorary Consultant Rheumatologist, University College London Hsopitals.

Neurology
Geraint Rees MRCP PhD, Wellcome Senior Clinical Fellow, Institute of Cognitive Neuroscience, University of London, London.

Psychiatry
Mo Zoha MB ChB MRCPsych, Consultant Psychiatrist, St Charles Hospital, London.

Basic Sciences

Best of Five

Questions

BASIC SCIENCES 'BEST OF FIVE' QUESTIONS

For each of the questions select the ONE most appropriate answer from the options provided.

1.1   You review a 54-year-old man with type-2 diabetes. He is currently managed with metformin 2g orally, twice daily and pioglitazone 45 mg daily. His BMI is 32. His blood results are haemoglobin (Hb) 14.0 g/dl, white cell count (WCC) 5.1 ×10^9/L, PLT 210 ×10^9/L, Na 140 mmol/l, K 4.9 mmol/l, Cr 120 μmol/l, Hb A$_{1c}$ 8.7%. He refuses insulin and you commence exenatide, a GLP-1 analogue. Which of the following fits best with the description of GLP-1?

    ☐ **A** It is produced by P-cells in the small intestine

    ☐ **B** It leads to increased production of glucagon

    ☐ **C** Excess leads to weight gain

    ☐ **D** It leads to improved secretion of insulin

    ☐ **E** Excess leads to accelerated β-cell death

1.2   A 56-year-old man presents to the oncology clinic. He has had a left nephrectomy for renal cell carcinoma. Histology has shown tumour up to the resection margin and regional lymph node involvement is suspected. His chest X-ray shows a large nodule consistent with a metastasis. Blood results, haemoglobin (Hb) 10.9 g/dl, white cell count (WCC) 6.1 ×10^9/L, PLT 140 ×10^9/L, Na 140 mmol/l, K 4.8 mmol/l, Cr 108 μmol/l. You elect to commence sunitinib therapy in this patient, the drug is a tyrosine kinase inhibitor. Which of the following fits best with the action of receptor tyrosine kinases?

    ☐ **A** They lead to sulphonation of proteins

    ☐ **B** They lead to phosphorylation of proteins

    ☐ **C** They commonly block signal transmission

    ☐ **D** Their substrate is ADP

    ☐ **E** Their substrate is cyclic AMP

1.3 A 35-year-old man presents to the cardiology clinic 2 weeks after being resuscitated from a cardiac arrest, which occurred while he was playing squash. You understand that his father and one brother have died suddenly in past years. On examination he looks normal and cardiovascular examination is unremarkable. His electrocardiogram (ECG) reveals a QTc of 0.48 ms. Which one of the following best describes the QT interval?

☐ **A** It is associated with depolarisation

☐ **B** QTc of 0.48 ms is within the normal range

☐ **C** Prolongation is associated with a reduced incidence of VT

☐ **D** Abnormalities in cardiac sodium channels may increase the QT interval

☐ **E** Amiodarone is the best treatment for QT prolongation complicated by cardiac arrest.

1.4 You review a 47-year-old man in the endocrine clinic who is overweight and has difficult to control blood pressure. He is currently taking ramipril 10 mg daily and amlodipine 10 mg daily. He has an unremarkable past medical history apart from a penchant for sweets, particularly licorice. His blood pressure (BP) is 165/100 mmHg and he looks slightly cushingoid. Blood tests, Na 140 mmol/l, K 3.8 mmol/l, Cr 100 μmol/l. Which of the following is the most likely cause of his presentation?

☐ **A** Simple obesity

☐ **B** Licorice excess

☐ **C** Conn syndrome

☐ **D** Cushing disease

☐ **E** Alcohol excess

Answers on pages 85–102

1.5 A 28-year-old woman presents with a pulmonary embolus after a 4-hour plane flight on her return from holiday. She had a history of deep vein thrombosis that was thought to have been related to inactivity after a ski-ing injury some 5 years earlier. Bloods, haemoglobin (Hb) 14.2 g/dl, white cell count (WCC) 6.1 ×10⁹/L, PLT 200 ×10⁹/L, Na 140 mmol/l, K 5.0 mmol/l, Cr 105 μmol/l, PT 17s, APPT 33s, protein C 40% of normal. You diagnose protein C deficiency, which of the following is most true of protein C deficiency?

- ☐ **A** Protein C is a pro-coagulant
- ☐ **B** Protein C is pro-fibrinolytic
- ☐ **C** Protein C has anti-inflammatory activity
- ☐ **D** Homozygous protein C deficiency usually presents from the age of 5 years
- ☐ **E** Protein C deficiency is more common in women

1.6 A 57-year-old woman presents to the clinic with difficult to manage diabetes, diarrhoea and weight loss. She also complains of a migrating rash, which begins as maculopapular ringed lesions and blisters that burst after a few days. This occurs most commonly on the feet and hands, forearms, buttocks and groin area. Investigations, haemoglobin (Hb) 12.0 g/dl, PLT 190 ×10⁹/L, white cell count (WCC) 5.4 ×10⁹/L, glucose 12.1 mmol/l, glucagon 1200 ng/l. Which of the following fits best with the action of glucagon?

- ☐ **A** It reduces secretion of catecholamines
- ☐ **B** It increases urinary sodium retention
- ☐ **C** It stimulates hepatic glucose output
- ☐ **D** Pancreatic glucagon has 31 amino acids
- ☐ **E** Glucagonomas are associated with MEN-2

1.7 A 65-year-old man with chronic obstructive pulmonary disease (COPD) presents to the clinic for review. He has been diagnosed with chronic bronchitis some years earlier and is managed with high dose combination steroid and long-acting beta-2-agonist therapy. Arterial blood gases reveal pH 7.32, $p(O_2)$ 7.3, $p(CO_2)$ 6.8, HCO_3 30. Which of the following fits best with this case?

☐ **A** His renal carbonic acid secretion is likely to be decreased

☐ **B** Renal bicarbonate reabsorption is increased

☐ **C** He has an acute respiratory acidosis

☐ **D** He has a metabolic alkalosis

☐ **E** Renal compensation of respiratory acidosis occurs within 24 h

1.8 A 74-year-old man is brought to the GP by his wife. She has noticed that he is increasingly tired and lethargic and complains of some numbness in his feet. Blood tests reveal haemoglobin (Hb) 10.0 g/dl, mean corpuscular volume (MCV) 106 fL, white cell count (WCC) 4.5 $\times 10^9$/L, PLT 110 $\times 10^9$/L, K 4.9 mmol/l, Na 140 mmol/l, Cr 140 μmol/l, TSH 1.2 mU/L, intrinsic factor antibody +. Which of the following fits best with this clinical picture?

☐ **A** Serum vitamin B_{12} levels are likely to be elevated

☐ **B** Intrinsic factor allows for vitamin B_{12} absorbtion in the jejunum

☐ **C** Bacterial overgrowth is the most likely cause here

☐ **D** Oral vitamin B_{12} supplementation is the treatment of choice

☐ **E** Autoimmune thyroid disease occurs more commonly in patients with this condition

1.9 A 56-year-old man presents with central crushing chest pain, sweating and hypotension. He has a history of hypertension and type-2 diabetes. Blood tests reveal an elevated CK of 760. His electrocardiogram (ECG) reveals tall R waves in V1 and V2 and deep ST depression in leads V1–V3. Which of the following fits best with the area of the heart that is affected?

☐ **A** The inferior area

☐ **B** The anterior area

☐ **C** The lateral area

☐ **D** The apical area

☐ **E** The posterior area

Answers on pages 85–102

1.10 A 42-year-old rough sleeper is admitted to the Emergency Unit, he is drowsy and intoxicated. He complains of blurred vision and is vomiting profusely. His respiratory rate is 28. His blood glucose is measured at 2.8 mmol/l, pH 7.21, $p(O_2)$ 8.9, $p(CO_2)$ 3.5, Na 140 mmol/l, K 4.5 mmol/l, Cl 105 mmol/l, bicarbonate 17 mmol/l. A friend enquires of his health and tells you that he has been drinking some methanol. Which of the following fits best with this case?

☐ **A** Toxicity is due to accumulation of acetic acid

☐ **B** Formaldehyde accumulates in methanol toxicity

☐ **C** Ethanol is not an acceptable treatment for methanol toxicity

☐ **D** Up-regulation of alcohol dehydrogenase is the key objective of treatment

☐ **E** A level of 200 mg/dl is rarely fatal

1.11 A 21-year-old Swedish woman is admitted to the Emergency Room complaining of abdominal pain. This has been her third admission over the past year. Her only medication of note is the combined oral contraceptive pill. On this occasion she is also noted to be hypertensive and tachycardic, there are no skin rashes. Bloods: haemoglobin (Hb) 13.1 g/dl, white cell count (WCC) 9.9×10^9/L, PLT 160×10^9/L, Na 130 mmol/l, K 5.0 mmol/l, Cr 105 µmol/l. Urinary coporphobilinogen elevated, stool porphyrins mildly elevated. Which of the following is true of this condition?

☐ **A** The condition is most common in patients of African descent

☐ **B** It occurs due to a defect in haem breakdown

☐ **C** It occurs due to a defect in haem synthesis

☐ **D** A skin rash is common

☐ **E** There is a male preponderance

1.12 A 26-year-old woman presents to the clinic for her 14-week pregnancy check. She is very well but the nurse notices that her urine contains 1+ of glucose on dipstick testing. A fasting plasma glucose is arranged and this is 4.1 mmol/l, she has an oral glucose tolerance test that is normal. Which of the following fits best with this case?

☐ **A** She is at increased risk of type-2 diabetes later in life

☐ **B** Her presentation is likely to be due to increased insulin resistance

☐ **C** A mutation coding for SGLT-1 is most likely to be responsible

☐ **D** A mutation in the *SLC5A2* gene may be the cause

☐ **E** She is likely to suffer from hypertension

1.13 A 42-year-old woman presents to the medical services while on a walking holiday in the USA. She had been walking 2 days earlier through a forested region. She is complaining of a rash affecting her forearms that appeared a few hours earlier, she thinks that she may have brushed against some ivy. On examination she has an oedematous erythaematous rash affecting both forearms with formation of small vesicles. Which of the following is most likely to be true of this case?

☐ **A** The likely cause is an immediate hypersensitivity reaction

☐ **B** Release of IL-1 is not related to development of symptoms

☐ **C** Release of IL-2 is unlikely to be increased in the area of the rash

☐ **D** IL-6 is involved in the inflammatory pathway

☐ **E** B-lymphocytes are strongly linked to the development of the rash

Answers on pages 85–102

1.14   A 19-year-old student presents to the university health service
        complaining of flu-like symptoms and that he is off his food. On
        examination he is mildly jaundiced. On further questioning he admits to
        two other episodes of jaundice in the past. Blood results reveal bilirubin
        82 μmol/l, alanine aminotransferase (ALT) 22 u/L, alkaline phosphatase
        45 u/l, albumin 40 g/L, haemoglobin (Hb) 14.0 g/dl, white cell count
        (WCC) 4.5 ×10^9/L, PLT 180 ×10^9/L. The GP institutes a trial of
        barbiturates, which resolves his jaundice. Which of the following is true
        of his condition?

    ☐   A   It is due to a rise in conjugated bilirubin
    ☐   B   Viral infection is the most likely cause
    ☐   C   Glucuronyl transferase defect is the most likely cause
    ☐   D   It is commoner in women
    ☐   E   It is associated with increased risk of cirrhosis

1.15   You review a 56-year-old man with type-2 diabetes. His Hb A_{1c} is 7.5%
        on metformin 2 g/day. You elect to commence him on pioglitazone, a
        PPAR-γ agonist. Which of the following is true of PPAR-γ agonists?

    ☐   A   They are associated with elevations in HDL cholesterol
    ☐   B   They promote de-differentiation of adipocytes
    ☐   C   They lead to a rise in free-fatty acids
    ☐   D   They lead to profound decreases in hepatic fat
    ☐   E   They are a primary treatment for dyslipidaemia

1.16   A 39-year-old man is referred to the Neurology Department with a
        history of chorea, ataxia and cognitive decline. He is subsequently
        diagnosed with Huntington disease. Which one of the following
        statements regarding this disorder is correct?

    ☐   A   It is autosomal recessively inherited
    ☐   B   All daughters of affected men are affected, but none of their sons
    ☐   C   All his offspring have a 50% chance of inheriting the disease
    ☐   D   There is no male-to-male transmission
    ☐   E   It is caused by a mitochondrial DNA mutation

Answers on pages 85–102   9

1.17   A 17-year-old boy presents with a history of learning difficulties, behavioural problems, dysarthria and arthropathy. On examination, he has a marked tremor and Kayser–Fleischer corneal rings. He is investigated and a diagnosis of Wilson disease is made. Which one of the following statements regarding this disorder is correct?

☐ **A**   The gene is located on chromosome 6

☐ **B**   If an affected individual marries an unaffected individual 50% of the children will be carriers

☐ **C**   Affected men can only have normal sons and carrier daughters

☐ **D**   Affected cases are usually mans carrying the gene or (rarely) homozygous women

☐ **E**   When both parents carry the gene each of their offspring has a 1 in 4 (25%) chance of being affected and a 50% chance of being a carrier

1.18   A 29-year-old woman is admitted to the Emergency Department with a history of headache, photophobia, drowsiness and seizures. On examination she is pyrexial and confused. She has photophobia and neck stiffness. Computed tomography (CT) head scan suggests some temporal lobe swelling is present. No haemorrhage, infarct or mass lesion is seen. You perform a lumbar puncture and send off her cerebrospinal fluid (CSF) for MC&S, Gram stain, protein, glucose and virology. You are concerned she may have meningoencephalitis and ask the labs to do herpes simplex virus (HSV) PCR. You start her on intravenous aciclovir, ceftriaxone and benzylpenicillin and admit her to the Intensive Care Unit (ITU). Which one of the following statements regarding the polymerase chain reaction (PCR) is correct?

☐ **A**   It occurs at 40 °C

☐ **B**   It uses heat-labile DNA polymerase derived from *Thermus aquaticus*

☐ **C**   It can be used to amplify RNA directly

☐ **D**   It allows specific DNA sequences to be amplified from a single cell

☐ **E**   It involves cleavage of DNA with restriction enzymes, gel electrophoresis then visualisation on an autoradiograph following hybridisation with a specific DNA or RNA probe

Answers on pages 85–102

1.19 **A 22-year-old woman is admitted to the Emergency Department following a paracetamol overdose. She has also slashed her left wrist, severing the median nerve. Which one of the following signs would be consistent with this injury?**

☐ **A** Wasting and paralysis of the hypothenar muscles of the left hand

☐ **B** Loss of sensation over the palmar aspect of the left little finger

☐ **C** Paralysis of the intrinsic hand muscles (apart from the lateral two lumbricals) on the left

☐ **D** Wrist drop

☐ **E** Paralysis of the thenar muscles, ie opponens pollicis, abductor pollicis brevis and flexor pollicis brevis

1.20 **A 55-year-old man is a patient on the Neurology Ward. He has noticed some deterioration in his vision lately. On examination of his visual fields he has a left homonymous superior quadrantanopia. Which one of the following is the most likely cause?**

☐ **A** Pituitary tumour compressing the optic chiasma

☐ **B** A lesion in the right parietal lobe

☐ **C** Thrombotic stroke affecting the posterior cerebral artery distribution

☐ **D** Temporal lobe lesion

☐ **E** Optic neuritis

1.21 **A female patient presents with galactorrhoea. Which one of the following medications would be most likely to cause this?**

☐ A Tamoxifen

☐ B Co-careldopa

☐ C Cyclizine

☐ D Bromocriptine

☐ E Metoclopramide

1.22 A 65-year-old man who has been attending the Cardiology Clinic presents with increasing shortness of breath on exertion, a reduced appetite and skin discoloration. His investigations are as follows: haemoglobin 13 g/dl, WCC 7×10^9/l, platelets 190×10^9/l, sodium 135 mmol/l, potassium 4.1 mmol/l, urea 8.0 mmol/l, creatinine 100 μmol/l, aspartate aminotransferase (AST) 160 U/l, ALP 180 U/l, albumin 39 g/l, bilirubin 48 μmol/l, FT_4 24 pmol/l, TSH 0.2 mU/l. Pulmonary function tests (PFTs):

- actual predicted
- FEV_1 2.8 l 4.0 l
- FVC 3.1 l 5.0 l
- FEV_1/FVC ratio – 90%
- TLCO 0.7 1.6

Echocardiography shows an enlarged left atrium and a normal-sized left ventricle with good function and normal valves. Which of the following provides the best explanation for this patient's presentation?

- ☐ A Congestive cardiac failure (CCF)
- ☐ B Chest infection
- ☐ C Hyperthyroidism
- ☐ D Hereditary haemochromatosis
- ☐ E Amiodarone toxicity

1.23 Which one of the following would be most likely to lead to these results: sodium 137 mmol/l, potassium 5.0 mmol/l, urea 5.2 mmol/l, creatinine 95 μmol/l, glucose 1.9 mmol/l?

- ☐ **A** Polycystic ovarian syndrome
- ☐ **B** Haemochromatosis
- ☐ **C** Prednisolone treatment
- ☐ **D** Metformin treatment
- ☐ **E** Pituitary insufficiency

Answers on pages 85–102

1.24   A 22-year-old woman is admitted to the Emergency Department. Her plasma biochemistry is as follows: sodium 138 mmol/l, potassium 4.0 mmol/l, urea 5.0 mmol/l, creatinine 100 μmol/l, bicarbonate 18 mmol/l, chloride 105 mmol/l, glucose 5.0 mmol/l, plasma osmolality 307 mOsmol/kg. Which one of the following is most likely to have caused these results?

☐ **A** Type-2 renal tubular acidosis (RTA)

☐ **B** Addison disease

☐ **C** Aspirin overdose

☐ **D** Conn syndrome

☐ **E** Ethanol toxicity

1.25   A 36-year-old man is referred to the Rheumatology Clinic with a ten-year history of worsening lower back pain. Over the last year he has noticed pain in both knees. He also complains that his sweat is dark and stains his clothing. He has no history of rashes, alopecia, mouth or genital ulcers or diarrhoea. He did not complain of any eye problems. He had dysuria after a trip to Amsterdam at the age of 20 but this cleared up after treatment with oxytetracycline. He had no other PMH of note. On examination, abnormal pigmentation of his ears and sclerae is noted. He has lost his lumbar lordosis and lumbar spine flexion is reduced. His knee joints are swollen, with bilateral effusions. Examination of the rest of the musculoskeletal system is normal, as are cardiovascular, respiratory, gastrointestinal and neurological examinations. His investigations show the following: haemoglobin 13.5 g/dl, white cell count (WCC) 5×10^9/l, platelets 200×10^9/l, ESR 30 mm/h, corrected calcium 2.3 mmol/l, phosphate 0.8 mmol/l, alkaline phosphatase 90 U/l, albumin 40 g/l, glucose 3.8 mmol/l. X-rays reveal loss of lumbar lordosis and intervertebral disc calcification. Urinalysis shows glucose ++, no protein. Which one of the following is the most likely diagnosis?

☐ **A** Ankylosing spondylitis

☐ **B** Alkaptonuria (ochronosis)

☐ **C** Haemochromatosis

☐ **D** Osteoarthritis

☐ **E** Reiter syndrome

1.26   A 30-year-old woman presents with left loin pain. Her only other history is that of two vertebral crush fractures. Her investigations are: urinalysis blood +++, pH 7, serum sodium 135 mmol/l, potassium 2.8 mmol/l, urea 5.7 mmol/l, creatinine 107 μmol/l, chloride 115 mmol/l, bicarbonate 9 mmol/l. What is the most likely underlying diagnosis?

☐ **A**   Renal calculus

☐ **B**   Diabetic ketoacidosis (DKA)

☐ **C**   Type-1 (distal) renal tube acidosis (RTA)

☐ **D**   Urinary tract infection (UTI)

☐ **E**   Type-2 (proximal) RTA

1.27   You review a male patient with recently diagnosed liver cirrhosis. A liver screen has been done, which suggests chronic hepatitis C infection. Which one of the following statements regarding hepatitis C liver disease is true?

☐ **A**   Hepatitis C is a DNA virus

☐ **B**   Chronic liver disease occurs in 50–80% of those infected

☐ **C**   Interferon–γ [AQ]results in clearance of the virus in 90% of patients

☐ **D**   Fulminant hepatitis is common

☐ **E**   Transmission is usually faecal–oral

1.28   A 32-year-old man has hepatitis B. Which one of the following statements is true of this disease?

☐ **A**   The virus only infects hepatocytes

☐ **B**   80% of those infected develop chronic hepatitis B infection

☐ **C**   IgG HBcAb indicates previous infection, now cleared

☐ **D**   Blood levels of HBeAg correlate with infectivity

☐ **E**   Patients who are immunodeficient are more likely to develop fulminant hepatic failure than those who are immunocompetent

Answers on pages 85–102

1.29   You have joined Médecins Sans Frontières and have been posted to tropical Africa. One of your patients, a 19-year-old woman, presents with a sore throat, malaise and anorexia. On examination she has a low-grade fever, cervical lymphadenopathy and a bluish-white membrane covering her pharynx. Eleven days later her voice assumes a nasal quality and fluid regurgitates through her nose. Which one of the following statements regarding her diagnosis is correct?

☐ A   The causative organism is an invasive aerobic Gram-negative rod

☐ B   She is likely to have polio

☐ C   Treatment should only be started when there is laboratory confirmation of the diagnosis

☐ D   Treatment with antitoxin is unhelpful

☐ E   Severe complications occur due to the production of an exotoxin that inhibits protein synthesis

1.30   A 50-year-old man is admitted to the Emergency Department. His arterial blood gases are: pH 7.23, p_a (O_2) 7.0 kPa, p_a (CO_2) 8.1 kPa. Which one of the following would be most likely to produce these results?

☐ A   Pulmonary haemorrhage

☐ B   Pulmonary embolism

☐ C   Pneumothorax

☐ D   An overdose of diazepam

☐ E   Asthma

1.31   You are involved in running a hypertension-screening programme in your local area. Two thousand people, aged 30–80 years, are screened. Both the mean and the median of the systolic blood pressure distribution are approximately 145 mmHg and the standard deviation is 22 mmHg. Which one of the following statements is correct?

☐ A   5% of the subjects will have a systolic blood pressure greater than 189 mmHg

☐ B   Approximately 95% of the subjects have systolic blood pressures between 101 and 189 mmHg

☐ C   Approximately 68% of the subjects have systolic blood pressures between 101 and 189 mmHg

☐ D   99% of the observations lie within 2.6 standard errors of the mean

☐ E   The distribution is asymmetric

1.32 **A new oral hypoglycaemic is administered to patients with type-2 diabetes in a clinical trial. Which one of the following statements is correct?**

☐ **A** A fall in plasma glucose with a probability value of $P > 0.05$ would indicate that the drug has a significant effect

☐ **B** Parametrical tests should be used on data that has a skewed distribution

☐ **C** The statistical significance of the fall in blood glucose may be analysed by a paired Student's *t*-test

☐ **D** If the P value $= 0.01$, 1 in 20 studies would be expected to show a significant effect of the drug on blood glucose by chance alone

☐ **E** In a single-blind study neither the researcher nor the patient knows to which treatment the patient has been randomised

1.33 **Hormones are capable of acting at distant sites via specific, high-affinity receptors. Concerning hormone action, which one of the following statements is true?**

☐ **A** ACTH receptors are coupled to G proteins

☐ **B** Cortisol binds to the mineralocorticoid receptor

☐ **C** Insulin acts by causing dimerisation of two subunits of the insulin receptor and stimulating adenylate cyclase

☐ **D** PAR alpha binds to the thiazolidine group of drugs

☐ **E** Thyroid hormone binds to a membrane receptor

1.34 **In thyrotoxicosis, appropriate management depends on the aetiology and associated pathologies. Which of the following statements is true?**

☐ **A** Carbimazole is contraindicated in pregnancy

☐ **B** Graves disease is associated with myasthenia gravis

☐ **C** Graves ophthalmopathy requires high-dose steroid treatment

☐ **D** Radioactive iodine improves exophthalmos in Graves disease

☐ **E** Toxic multi-nodular goitre may go into long-term remission following a course of carbimazole

Answers on pages 85–102

1.35 **In the clinical evaluation of gynaecomastia which one of the following underlying diagnoses is unlikely?**

☐ **A** Amiodarone

☐ **B** Klinefelter syndrome

☐ **C** Renal failure

☐ **D** Spironolactone

☐ **E** Testicular malignancy

1.36 **In the management of acromegaly which one of the following statements is correct?**

☐ **A** 90% of patients respond to long-acting somatostatin analogue treatment

☐ **B** Diabetes mellitus occurs in <5% of patients

☐ **C** Hypercholesterolaemia is common

☐ **D** Patients with pituitary microadenomas can be cured in 50% of cases

☐ **E** Suprasellar extension prevents a trans-sphenoidal surgical approach

1.37 **Concerning monoclonal antibodies which one of the following statements is not true?**

☐ **A** They are used to limit transplant rejection

☐ **B** They are made using human B lymphocytes

☐ **C** They can be used to activate T lymphocytes in vitro

☐ **D** They can be used to detect proteins in histological sections

☐ **E** They can be used to measure hormones in blood

1.38 **Which one of the following is a characteristic of mitochondrial diseases?**

☐ **A** They cause hypothyroidism

☐ **B** They cause ketoacidosis

☐ **C** They cause 'ragged red' fibres in skeletal muscle

☐ **D** They involve the renal tubule

☐ **E** They are paternally inherited

1.39 **Concerning genetic anticipation:**
- ☐ **A** It is characteristic of neurofibromatosis type-1
- ☐ **B** It is not seen with fragile-X syndrome
- ☐ **C** It refers to earlier diagnosis due to improved awareness
- ☐ **D** It occurs in Turner syndrome
- ☐ **E** It results from amplification of triplet repeats within genes

1.40 **Concerning the regulation of gene expression, which one of the following statements is correct?**
- ☐ **A** Introns are not transcribed into mRNA
- ☐ **B** Mammalian mRNA tends to be polycistronic
- ☐ **C** Mutations in the DNA sequence encoding a gene always result in changes in the amino acid sequence of the resulting protein
- ☐ **D** RNA polymerase II gives rise to protein encoding mRNA
- ☐ **E** The majority of cellular RNA is mRNA

1.41 **Tumour necrosis factor-α:**
- ☐ **A** Activates the nuclear factor kappa B (NFκB) transcription factor
- ☐ **B** Binds a single, specific receptor
- ☐ **C** Inhibits expression of interleukin-1 (IL-1)
- ☐ **D** Is useful treatment for rheumatoid arthritis
- ☐ **E** Leads to enhanced insulin sensitivity

1.42 **In rheumatoid arthritis, which one of the following is true?**
- ☐ **A** Association of seropositivity with HLA-DR1
- ☐ **B** Concordance rate of >60% for identical twins
- ☐ **C** Peak incidence in the third decade
- ☐ **D** Progression from predominantly small peripheral joint disease to involve more proximal, larger joints
- ☐ **E** Sacroiliac joint disease is common

Answers on pages 85–102

1.43   **In polymyalgia rheumatica:**

   ☐ **A** Electromyography (EMG) studies detect a typical abnormality

   ☐ **B** Night sweats and fever make the diagnosis unlikely

   ☐ **C** Half of patients are aged less than 60 years

   ☐ **D** Patients have a characteristic reduction in circulating $CD8^+$ T lymphocytes

   ☐ **E** The response to prednisolone is helpful in diagnosis

1.44   **The HLA-B27 molecule is:**

   ☐ **A** A class II major histocompatibility antigen

   ☐ **B** Expressed on antigen-presenting dendritic cells

   ☐ **C** Found in 50% of Whites with ankylosing spondylitis

   ☐ **D** Over-represented in Crohn disease

   ☐ **E** Over-represented in Whipple disease

1.45   **Systemic lupus erythaematosus (SLE) is a systemic inflammatory disease. Which one of the following statements is true concerning SLE?**

   ☐ **A** 15% have Raynaud's phenomenon

   ☐ **B** C-reactive protein is a useful marker of disease activity

   ☐ **C** It is less common in Klinefelter syndrome

   ☐ **D** High frequencies of disease are seen in women of Chinese ancestry

   ☐ **E** The skin is affected in < 50% of cases

1.46   **Concerning urinary sediment, which one of the following is correct?**

   ☐ **A** Less than 100 white cells per ml is normal

   ☐ **B** Cystine crystals are often found in normal urine

   ☐ **C** Hyaline casts consist of Tamm–Horsfall protein

   ☐ **D** Oxalate crystals in the urine suggest renal disease

   ☐ **E** Red cells always indicate renal tract disease

Answers on pages 85–102

1.47 **Patients with renal failure may require drug treatment in addition to haemodialysis. Which one of the following drugs is dialysed by haemodialysis?**

☐ **A** Aciclovir

☐ **B** Erythromycin

☐ **C** Propranolol

☐ **D** Vancomycin

☐ **E** Warfarin

1.48 **In the evaluation of a patient with raised urea and creatinine, pre-renal failure is unlikely if there is:**

☐ **A** Decreased pulmonary wedge pressure

☐ **B** Postural hypotension

☐ **C** Urine osmolality > 500 mOsm/l

☐ **D** Urine sodium > 20 mmol/l

☐ **E** Urine to plasma urea ratio of > 8

1.49 **Concerning adult polycystic kidney disease, which one of the following is true?**

☐ **A** 10% of affected patients will also have hepatic cysts

☐ **B** Abdominal pain is a common presenting feature

☐ **C** It has autosomal recessive inheritance

☐ **D** Generally results in end-stage renal failure in the third decade

☐ **E** Spontaneous haematuria is unusual

1.50 **Concerning acid–base function of the kidney, which one of the following statements is not true?**

☐ **A** > 80% of all filtered bicarbonate ions are actively recovered

☐ **B** In distal renal tubular acidosis (RTA type-1) there is normal anion gap, metabolic acidosis and urinary pH > 5.5

☐ **C** Nephrocalcinosis suggests type-1 or distal RTA

☐ **D** Proximal renal tubular acidosis is usually an inherited condition

☐ **E** The proximal nephron actively secretes hydrogen ions, in contrast to the distal nephron

Answers on pages 85–102

1.51   With regard to human immunodeficiency virus (HIV):

☐ **A** CD8 cells become depleted as disease progresses

☐ **B** HIV-1 and HIV-2 are closely related and cause similar disease progression

☐ **C** HIV gains entry to the cell via the TNF receptor

☐ **D** It is a lentivirus

☐ **E** The HIV genome contains circular DNA

1.52   Concerning pneumococcal disease:

☐ **A** Pneumococcal meningitis is associated with similar mortality rates to meningococcal meningitis in industrialised countries

☐ **B** Pneumococcal otitis media is usually associated with neutrophil leucocytosis

☐ **C** Pneumococcal pneumonia shows no seasonal variation in temperate countries

☐ **D** *Pneumococcus* is a Gram-negative organism

☐ **E** Sickle cell disease predisposes to pneumococcal infection and antibiotic prophylaxis is ineffective

1.53   Concerning herpes simplex virus infection, which one of the following is correct?

☐ **A** 10% of herpes encephalitis cases are due to reactivation of virus

☐ **B** Antibody titres are helpful in making management decisions

☐ **C** It is caused by a single-stranded DNA virus

☐ **D** Herpes meningitis is a relatively benign condition in adults

☐ **E** Precedes 50% of all cases of erythaema multiforme

1.54   Concerning meningococcal disease, which one of the following statements is untrue?

☐ **A** Haemorrhagic skin lesions are a late feature of septicaemia

☐ **B** Identification of Gram-positive diplococci on lumbar puncture suggests meningococcal meningitis

☐ **C** Meningococcaemia is associated with neutrophilia

☐ **D** Rifampicin eradicates nasal carriage in fewer than 30% of contacts

☐ **E** Transmission is usually by respiratory droplet

Answers on pages 85–102

1.55 **Which one of the following is true of Marfan syndrome?**

☐ **A** Aortic dissection is a recognised complication

☐ **B** Mutations in the collagen gene are typical

☐ **C** New mutations in the gene are rare

☐ **D** The inheritance pattern is X-linked dominant

☐ **E** The mutations generally occur at the same position within the gene

Infectious Diseases

Best of Five

Questions

INFECTIOUS DISEASES 'BEST OF FIVE' QUESTIONS

For each of the questions select the ONE most appropriate answer from the options provided.

2.1 A 22-year-old man presents to the Emergency Room complaining of fever and abdominal pain, diarrhoea and a cough productive of blood-stained sputum. He has recently returned from South-East Asia and is HIV positive. On further questioning, he reports night sweats, worsening dyspnoea on exertion and some weight loss. Examination reveals a temperature of 38.9 °C, and a tachycardia of 105, he is cachectic and drowsy but can be roused relatively easily. Inspiratory and expiratory crackles are heard over the right anterior chest. Blood investigations: haemoglobin (Hb) 8.1 g/dl, mean corpuscular volume (MCV) 69.1 fl, white cell count (WCC) 4.9 ×10⁹/L, platelets (PLT) 200 ×10⁹/L, CD4 10 ×10⁶/L, alkaline phosphate 301 U/l, aspartate aminotransferase (AST) 60 U/l, LDH 700 iu/l, chest X-ray (CXR) – right-sided pulmonary infiltrates, pH 7.46, $p(CO_2)$ 3.4, $p(O_2)$ 7.9. Which one of the following is the most likely diagnosis?

☐ **A** *Mycobacterium avium intracellulare*

☐ **B** Histoplasmosis

☐ **C** *Cryptococcus*

☐ **D** Lymphoma

☐ **E** *Mycoplasma pneumoniae*

2.2   A 31-year-old woman who is 6 months' pregnant presents to the
       Emergency department feeling unwell. She has returned to the UK from
       Kenya where she accompanies her husband who works for the Embassy.
       Her complaint is of severe flu-like symptoms, with paroxysms of shaking
       chills, fevers and sweats. On examination she looks pale, is tachycardic
       with a pulse of 100, and her blood pressure (BP) is 100/70 mmHg.
       Investigations: haemoglobin (Hb) 9.2 g/dl, haptoglobins elevated, thick
       and thin blood-film malaria parasites identified, white cell count (WCC)
       12.1 ×10^9/L, platelets (PLT) 90 ×10^9/L, Na 140 mmol/l, K 5.4 mmol/l,
       Cr 150 µmol/l, bilirubin 190 µmol/l. Which one of the following is true
       when considering her condition?

☐ **A** Pregnant women are five times more likely to suffer from malaria

☐ **B** Malaria tends to be less severe in pregnancy

☐ **C** Quinidine is the best option for treatment

☐ **D** Primigravida women appear the most at risk from infection

☐ **E** Most prophylaxis options are contraindicated in pregnancy

2.3   A 25-year-old man presents to the Emergency Room with severe
       paroxysms of fever, sweating and rigors. Additionally he has arthralgia,
       myalgia and a cough. His symptoms began a few days ago. He has
       recently returned from a VSO project teaching in a school in Malawi. On
       examination, he is drowsy and looks very pale and unwell. He has a
       temperature of 39 °C and a blood pressure (BP) of 90/60 mmHg, his
       pulse is 100 and regular, he looks a little jaundiced. Investigations reveal:
       haemoglobin (Hb) 7.9 g/dl – raised MCV, white cell count (WCC)
       13.0 ×10^9/L, platelets (PLT) 85 ×10^9/L, elevated haptoglobins, thick and
       thin blood-film malaria parasites identified, Na 138 mmol/l,
       K 5.7 mmol/l, Cr 180 µmol/l. You elect to begin urgent drug therapy,
       which one of the following correctly fits with the mode of action of
       quinine?

☐ **A** It decreases pH in intracellular organelles

☐ **B** It increases pH in intracellular organelles and may interact with
          parasite DNA

☐ **C** It interferes with parasite ribosome activity

☐ **D** It binds to parasite DNA and may disrupt mitochondrial activity

☐ **E** It blocks entry of the parasite into erythrocytes

                                              Answers on pages 105–118

2.4   A 19-year-old builder comes to the clinic for review. He is concerned by the fact that he has developed a cluster of unsightly genital warts on his penis. On further questioning, he gives a history of unprotected sex with a number of female partners over the past two years. Investigations reveal: haemoglobin (Hb) 14.0 g/dl, white cell count (WCC) 8.0 ×10⁹/L, platelets (PLT) 301 ×10⁹/L, HIV negative, hepatitis B negative, syphilis serology negative. Which one of the following is true of his condition?

    ☐   **A**   Unprotected sex with a female partner will greatly increase her chance of developing cervical carcinoma

    ☐   **B**   Biopsy is necessary to confirm the diagnosis

    ☐   **C**   Human papillomavirus (HPV) subtypes 6 and 11 commonly cause this infection

    ☐   **D**   A vaccine does not currently exist with activity against genital warts

    ☐   **E**   Spontaneous regression of the warts is very uncommon

2.5   A 20-year-old student is brought to the Emergency Room by his flatmates. He has suffered from a sore throat and flu-like symptoms for the past few days and suddenly deteriorated. They found him in bed, drowsy and moaning, complaining of a severe headache and neck stiffness. On examination, his blood pressure is 100/50 mmHg, with a pulse of 100, his temperature is 39 °C. He has a haemorrhagic rash. There are marked signs of meningism. Investigations reveal: haemoglobin (Hb) 12.1 g/dl, white cell count (WCC) 15.2 ×10⁹/L, platelets (PLT) 95 ×10⁹/L, Na 140 mmol/l, K 5.4 mmol/l, Cr 145 μmol/l, lumbar puncture: Gram-negative diplococci seen. Which one of the following is true of this condition?

    ☐   **A**   The bacteria are always sensitive to penicillin

    ☐   **B**   Epidemics in young people were often due to the 'C' type

    ☐   **C**   A highly effective vaccine exists for the 'B' type

    ☐   **D**   Infection is commoner in the first few months of life

    ☐   **E**   Cotrimoxazole is commonly used for prophylaxis

2.6 A 27-year-old man who has been to Bratislava for a friend's stag party presents to the sexually transmitted diseases clinic 4 weeks later. He has noticed a firm, painless lump on his glans penis for over a week. There are also swollen lymph nodes in the groin. On examination, he has a raised, firm ulcer on the glans penis and inguinal lymphadenopathy. Investigations reveal: haemoglobin (Hb) 13.9 g/dl, white cell count (WCC) 7.2 ×10⁹/L, platelets (PLT) 205 ×10⁹/L, venereal disease research laboratory (VDRL) positive, Na 139 mmol/l, K 4.0 mmol/l, Cr 103 μmol/l. Which one of the following is true of the condition?

☐ **A** Penicillin im is the treatment of choice

☐ **B** Patients may require lifelong treatment with aciclovir

☐ **C** The incidence of new cases of this infection in the UK is decreasing

☐ **D** Tracing of sexual contacts is not required

☐ **E** This man should not be offered an HIV test

2.7 A 22-year-old man presents to the sexually transmitted diseases clinic complaining of an itchy, red and painful glans penis. He has also noticed a whitish discharge. There is a history of type 1 diabetes, controlled with insulin, also of note is that he had unprotected sex around 3 weeks earlier. Investigations reveal: haemoglobin (Hb) 13.8 g/dl, white cell count (WCC) 5.4 ×10⁹/L, platelets (PLT) 230 ×10⁹/L, Hb A₁c 9%, Na 139 mmol/l, K 4.0 mmol/l, Cr 80 μmol/l. Which one of the following is the most likely diagnosis?

☐ **A** *Candida albicans*

☐ **B** Reiter syndrome

☐ **C** *Gardnerella vaginalis*

☐ **D** *Treponema pallidum*

☐ **E** Lichen sclerosus

Answers on pages 105–118

2.8   A 26-year-old woman presents to the clinic complaining of copious amounts of fish-smelling vaginal discharge, which is a homogenous grey/yellow discharge. She has been troubled by this for a few months, and is continuously washing to try to get herself clean. There is no recent history of unprotected sexual intercourse. Investigations: haemoglobin (Hb) 13.0 mmHg, white cell count (WCC) 4.5 $\times 10^9$/L, platelets (PLT) 350 $\times 10^9$/L, Na 139 mmol/l, K 5.0 mmol/l, Cr 80 μmol/l, vaginal pH 4.8, amine-like smell. Clue cells present on microscopy. Which one of the following is the most likely diagnosis?

- ☐ **A** *Candida albicans*
- ☐ **B** Bacterial vaginosis
- ☐ **C** *Trichomonas vaginalis*
- ☐ **D** *Chlamydia trachomatis*
- ☐ **E** *Neisseria gonorrhoeae*

2.9   A 32-year-old man presents to the HIV clinic for review. He has taken a number of combination therapies over the years, but you are concerned that his viral load has begun to rise. You elect to begin a treatment with maraviroc. Which one of the following is true of maraviroc?

- ☐ **A** It blocks binding to a receptor found predominantly on B cells
- ☐ **B** It is a reverse transcriptase inhibitor
- ☐ **C** It is a nucleoside analogue
- ☐ **D** Another member of the class has been terminated due to hepatotoxicity
- ☐ **E** The drug targets binding to the CCR4 receptor

2.10 You are working on an attachment with the VSO in Thailand and admit the son of a man who works at the poultry market. He is 12 years old. His temperature is 39 °C, with a pulse of 100, auscultation of the chest reveals coarse crackles and wheeze consistent with pneumonia. Investigations: haemoglobin (Hb) 13.9 g/dl, white cell count (WCC) 10.0 ×10^9/L, platelets (PLT) 290 ×10^9/L, Na 139 mmol/l, K 4.3 mmol/l, Cr 90 µmol/l, pH 7.32, $p(O_2)$ 7.6, $p(CO_2)$ 3.5. You are concerned about the possibility of H5N1. Which one of the following is true of the condition?

☐ **A** A high level of resistance to zanamivir has been identified

☐ **B** No resistance to oseltamivir has been identified

☐ **C** Human-to-human transmission is common

☐ **D** Close proximity to poultry is not thought to increase the risk of infection

☐ **E** The virus was first identified in Hong Kong

2.11 A 23-year-old woman presents to the GP complaining of left-sided pelvic pain and intermittent fever. She has also had bleeding after intercourse on two occasions. Her GP diagnosed recurrent urinary tract infections, but she has not really improved after a course of trimethoprim. Examination reveals cervical and adnexal tenderness and a mucopurulent cervical discharge. Investigations: haemoglobin (Hb) 13.8 g/dl, white cell count (WCC) 6.0 ×10^9/L, platelets (PLT) 298 ×10^9/L, Na 139 mmol/l, K 4.5 mmol/l, Cr 100 µmol/l. Which one of the following is the most likely diagnosis?

☐ **A** Cervical carcinoma

☐ **B** *Chlamydia trachomatis*

☐ **C** Trichomoniasis

☐ **D** *E. coli* urinary tract infection

☐ **E** Bacterial vaginosis

Answers on pages 105–118

2.12 A 42-year-old musician presents for review, he complains of increasing lethargy for the past 3–6 months, with nausea, anorexia and weight loss. On examination, he has signs of chronic liver disease with mild jaundice, spider naevi, loss of body hair and ascites. Investigations: haemoglobin (Hb) 11.1 g/dl, white cell count (WCC) 5.9 ×10^9/L, platelets (PLT) 195 ×10^9/L, alanine aminotransferase (ALT) 170 U/l, bilirubin 120 mmol/l, anti-HCV antibody positive, genotype 1 virus identified. Which one of the following is true of this condition?

☐ **A** Antiviral treatment for 6 months is usually sufficient

☐ **B** Genotype 1 accounts for between 40 and 80% of hepatitis C cases

☐ **C** Genotype 3 is found predominantly in Egypt

☐ **D** Liver biopsy commonly demonstrates macrophage infiltration

☐ **E** Hepatocellular carcinoma develops an average of 10 years after infection

2.13 A 26-year-old woman who is a known iv drug abuser presents to the antenatal clinic. She is 22 weeks' pregnant. You send off an antenatal screening batch of blood tests. Haemoglobin (Hb) 11.0 g/dl, white cell count (WCC) 6.1 ×10^9/L, platelets (PLT) 232 ×10^9/L, Na 139 mmol/l, K 4.3 mmol/l, Cr 90 μmol/l, alanine aminotransferase (ALT) 130 U/l, hepatitis B surface Ag +, hepatitis B envelope Ag positive, HIV negative. Which one of the following is true with respect to this case?

☐ **A** Acute hepatitis B is more severe in pregnancy

☐ **B** Chronic hepatitis B occurs in around 2% of pregnancies

☐ **C** The risk of transmission to the child is around 90%

☐ **D** 60% of cases of transmission to the child occur intrapartum

☐ **E** Immunisation is effective in reducing transmission rates by around 20%

2.14 **Which one of the following statements about the prion protein is true?**

☐ **A** Prion protein is encoded on the host genome

☐ **B** The amino acid sequence of the prion protein in variant Creutzfeldt–Jakob disease (vCJD) is the same as that in bovine spongiform encephalopathy

☐ **C** The risk of early or late onset of disease cannot be predicted

☐ **D** The infectivity of prion protein can be reduced by nucleases

☐ **E** Tonsillar biopsy can assist in the diagnosis of sporadic Creutzfeldt–Jakob disease

2.15 **A patient with HIV has a CD4 count of 25 × 10⁶ cells/l. It is likely that he will respond poorly to any vaccination, but which vaccine is absolutely contraindicated?**

☐ **A** Hepatitis B vaccine

☐ **B** Hepatitis A vaccine

☐ **C** Pneumococcal vaccine

☐ **D** Yellow fever vaccine

☐ **E** Rabies vaccine

2.16 **In the UK there is a legal duty on the attending physician to notify a number of infectious diseases to the Consultant in Communicable Disease Control. Other infections should be reported as a matter of good practice if there is a public health implication. Which one of the following infections is a legally notifiable disease?**

☐ **A** Brucellosis

☐ **B** Q fever

☐ **C** Legionnaires' disease

☐ **D** Lyme disease

☐ **E** Hepatitis C

Answers on pages 105–118

2.17 A 25-year-old Australian backpacker swam in Lake Malawi four months ago. He now has a peripheral blood eosinophilia and bloody diarrhoea. Which one of the following investigations is most likely to confirm the diagnosis?

☐ **A** Stool culture

☐ **B** Midnight blood sample for the presence of microfilaria

☐ **C** Amoebic serology

☐ **D** Rectal biopsy

☐ **E** Thick blood film for trypanosomes

2.18 A 50-year-old UK-born man has been on a walking safari in a game park in northern South Africa, never having previously been out of Europe. He presents seven days later with a fever and two black scabbing lesions on his legs. Two other people in his party of 20 also have a similar illness. What is the most appropriate treatment?

☐ **A** Co-amoxiclav

☐ **B** Doxycycline

☐ **C** Praziquantel

☐ **D** Sodium stibogluconate

☐ **E** Melarsoprol

2.19 A 30-year-old UK man who has had a regular sexual partner and no other partners over the previous two years presents with a urethral discharge and discomfort on passing urine. Clinical examination is unremarkable. Moderately abundant neutrophil polymorphs, but no organisms, are seen on the Gram stain of the urethral discharge. Which is the most likely causative organism?

☐ **A** *Treponema pallidum*

☐ **B** *Chlamydia trachomatis*

☐ **C** *Trichomonas vaginalis*

☐ **D** Herpes simplex

☐ **E** *Neisseria gonorrhoeae*

Answers on pages 105–118

2.20   A 20-year-old man arrives in the UK with a mosquito-borne illness. He is transferred to a specialist unit. The referral letter states that he has just arrived in the UK from India but you know that this travel history must be wrong. Which infection does he have?

☐ **A** *Wucheria bancrofti* filariasis

☐ **B** Japanese encephalitis

☐ **C** Dengue fever

☐ **D** Yellow fever

☐ **E** *Plasmodium vivax* malaria

2.21   A 17-year-old boy develops a sore throat with enlarged tonsils and generalised lymphadenopathy. A blood film shows an excess of atypical lymphocytes and a Paul–Bunnell test is strongly positive. Which one of the following is true?

☐ **A** The sore throat should be treated with co-amoxiclav

☐ **B** The atypical lymphocytes are activated B lymphocytes

☐ **C** The Paul–Bunnell test detects neutralising antibodies directed against Epstein–Barr virus

☐ **D** Tonsillar enlargement causing respiratory obstruction should be treated with ganciclovir

☐ **E** Persistent, uncontrolled infection can occur as an X-linked condition in males

2.22   A 54-year-old woman born in the mid-west USA and resident in the UK for the past 15 years (with her most recent visit back to the mid-west USA six months ago) develops an acute pneumonia. Two sets of blood cultures taken before the start of antibiotic treatment are negative. Which one of the following statements is most likely to be correct?

☐ **A** The causative agent is unlikely to be *Streptococcus pneumoniae*

☐ **B** Negative *Coxiella burnetii* serology taken on day 3 of the illness effectively excludes Q fever

☐ **C** Negative *Legionella* urinary antigen effectively excludes *Legionella*

☐ **D** The illness is highly unlikely to be acute pulmonary histoplasmosis

☐ **E** The presence of cold agglutinins is suggestive of *Mycoplasma* infection but it is a highly non-specific test

Answers on pages 105–118

2.23 A herdsman from the Middle East is admitted with a three-day history of fever shortly after his arrival in the UK. A zoonosis is suspected. His white blood cell count and platelet count are normal, but his C-reactive protein is elevated. A thick blood film stained with Giemsa stain does not show any parasites. Blood cultures become positive after five days' incubation. Which of the following is the most likely disease?

☐ **A** Brucellosis

☐ **B** Rift Valley fever (RVF)

☐ **C** Q fever

☐ **D** Sleeping sickness

☐ **E** Crimea Congo haemorrhagic fever (CCHF)

2.24 A patient with advanced AIDS, who has never travelled outside the UK, develops severe *Pneumocystis jiroveci* pneumonia and requires ventilation on the Intensive Care Unit (ICU). Blood cultures taken on days 10, 11 and 12 of the ICU stay all grow a fungus. Which is the most likely organism?

☐ **A** *Candida albicans*

☐ **B** *Aspergillus fumigatus*

☐ **C** *Pneumocystis jiroveci*

☐ **D** *Histoplasma capsulatum*

☐ **E** *Coccidioides immitis*

Answers on pages 105–118

2.25 **A previously fit 25-year-old man develops mild nausea two weeks into a course of treatment for smear-positive pulmonary tuberculosis. He has been prescribed correct doses of rifampicin, isoniazid, ethambutol and pyrazinamide. Full blood count, urea and electrolytes are normal. Alkaline phosphatase and serum bilirubin are normal. Alanine aminotransferase (ALT) is 153 U/l and aspartate transaminase (AST) is 160 U/l. A clotting screen is normal. What is the most appropriate course of action?**

☐ **A** Immediately stop all treatment and repeat liver function tests in one week, re-introducing treatment gradually when liver function tests are normal

☐ **B** Add pyridoxine to medication

☐ **C** Temporarily stop rifampicin, isoniazid and pyrazinamide, continuing the ethambutol

☐ **D** Continue all medication and repeat liver function tests in one week

☐ **E** Reduce the doses of rifampicin, isoniazid and pyrazinamide

2.26 **A 30-year-old woman from sub-Saharan Africa is diagnosed with advanced HIV (CD4 count 30 × 10⁶/l) and cervical lymph node and pulmonary tuberculosis. She is commenced on prophylactic co-trimoxizole, combination antiretroviral therapy and a standard quadruple antituberculous therapy (with doses adjusted correctly to compensate for drug interactions). Four weeks later she develops enlargement of her cervical lymph nodes, which ulcerate and discharge, shortness of breath and worsening of the pulmonary infiltrates on chest X-ray. What is the most likely explanation?**

☐ **A** Drug-resistant tuberculosis

☐ **B** Superadded infection with another opportunistic agent

☐ **C** Development of non-Hodgkin's lymphoma

☐ **D** Enhanced antimycobacterial immune reaction

☐ **E** Drug reaction

Answers on pages 105–118

2.27　A 35-year-old HIV-positive man has been taking zidovudine, lamivudine and nevirapine for the past two years, during which time he has been extremely well, with a CD4 count between 500 and 600 $\times$ 10⁶/l and HIV viral load less than 50 copies/ml. However his most recent blood test shows that his CD4 count has fallen to 150 $\times$ 10⁶/l and his HIV viral load has risen to 400,000 copies/ml. He comes to the clinic for the results of his blood tests. Which one of the following would you do at this clinic visit?

☐　**A**　Request sequencing of his HIV to look for mutations indicating resistance to antiretroviral drugs

☐　**B**　Add in a new antiretroviral agent that he has not had before

☐　**C**　Measure serum p24 antigen

☐　**D**　Change all his antiretroviral medication to a new combination

☐　**E**　Start prophylaxis against *Mycobacterium avium intracellulare* (MAI)

2.28　A 40-year-old woman, recently arrived in the UK from southern Sudan, presents with a two-month history of fever, marked hepatosplenomegaly and general wasting. Blood tests show her to be anaemic with a low platelet count, low albumin and high IgG. Repeated thin blood-film malaria are negative. What would be the next investigation of choice?

☐　**A**　Slit skin smear

☐　**B**　Bone marrow aspirate

☐　**C**　Thick blood film

☐　**D**　Liver biopsy

☐　**E**　Mantoux test

2.29　A 20-year-old leukaemic patient from the Middle East who has had a bone marrow transplant six weeks ago develops an anaemia, which responds to intravenous immunoglobulin. Which infectious agent is the likely cause?

☐　**A**　Parvovirus B19

☐　**B**　Cytomegalovirus

☐　**C**　Adenovirus

☐　**D**　*Mycobacterium tuberculosis*

☐　**E**　*Aspergillus fumigatus*

2.30 A 53-year-old man recently arrived from Ghana is diagnosed with *Plasmodium falciparum* malaria. A blood film shows that 40% of his red blood cells contain malaria parasites. His renal function is impaired and his conscious level is deteriorating. In addition to immediate resuscitation, which of the following is the first measure you would institute?

☐ **A** Atovaquone/proguanil combination therapy

☐ **B** Quinine

☐ **C** Chloroquine

☐ **D** Haemofiltration

☐ **E** Exchange transfusion

2.31 A 50-year-old man presents with a fever five days following his return from an eight-week holiday in Thailand. He is jaundiced but has no evidence of liver failure. He has marked renal impairment. He has a diminished cardiac output and an echocardiogram is consistent with a myocarditis. He subsequently develops pulmonary haemorrhage. What is the most likely diagnosis?

☐ **A** Scrub typhus (*Orienti tsutsugamushi*)

☐ **B** Leptospirosis

☐ **C** Typhoid fever

☐ **D** Melioidosis (*Burkholderia pseudomallei*)

☐ **E** Severe falciparum malaria

2.32 A 23-year-old man is investigated for hepatitis B virus (HBV) infection. Positive tests are found for hepatitis B surface antigen (HBsAg) and IgM antibodies to the core antigen (anti-HBc IgM) and a negative 'e' antigen (eAg). Which one of the following is the most likely clinical status?

☐ **A** Acute HBV infection

☐ **B** Chronic HBV carrier

☐ **C** Convalescence from acute HBV

☐ **D** None of the options

☐ **E** Previous immunisation against HBV

Answers on pages 105–118

2.33 **Which one of the following viral groups is least associated with haemorrhagic manifestations?**

☐ **A** Arbovirus

☐ **B** Arenavirus

☐ **C** Paramyxovirus

☐ **D** Picornavirus

☐ **E** Rotavirus

2.34 **When comparing Rhodesian and Gambian sleeping sickness, which one of the following statements is not true of both conditions?**

☐ **A** Central nervous system (CNS) abnormalities occur

☐ **B** Hepatosplenomegaly occurs

☐ **C** Humans are a recognised reservoir

☐ **D** Melarsoprol is effective treatment

☐ **E** The causative agent is *Trypanosoma brucei*

2.35 **In which one of the following malarial agents does a stage of exoerythrocytic schizogony definitely not occur?**

☐ **A** None of the options

☐ **B** *Plasmodium falciparum*

☐ **C** *Plasmodium malariae*

☐ **D** *Plasmodium ovale*

☐ **E** *Plasmodium vivax*

2.36   A 43-year-old male African immigrant, recently arrived in the UK, is
assessed by his general practitioner during registration. He has a
longstanding right hemiplegia and is blind in his left eye. There is a
history of recurrent pain and redness of the eyes with an occasional
exudative discharge. The general practitioner notes several small hard
subcutaneous nodules. Which one of the following is the most likely
diagnosis?

☐ **A** Cysticercosis

☐ **B** Filariasis

☐ **C** Hydatid disease

☐ **D** Schistosomiasis

☐ **E** Strongyloidiasis

2.37   Which one of the following is a high risk factor for contracting
Haemophilus?

☐ **A** Alcohol abuse

☐ **B** All of the options

☐ **C** Infancy and early childhood

☐ **D** Sickle-cell disease

☐ **E** Splenectomy

2.38   A 40-year-old British abattoir worker becomes systemically ill with
jaundice, microscopic haematuria and meningism. He is found to have
mild renal impairment, and haemolytic anaemia. There is no rash,
pharyngitis or lymphadenopathy. He has not travelled abroad. Which one
of the following is the most probable diagnosis?

☐ **A** Cholera

☐ **B** Coxsackievirus A

☐ **C** Infectious mononucleosis

☐ **D** Leptospirosis

☐ **E** Sporotrichosis

Answers on pages 105–118

2.39 **Which one of the following statements regarding staphylococcal and streptococcal infection is incorrect?**

- ☐ **A** Bacteraemia is uncommon in toxic shock syndrome
- ☐ **B** Group A *Streptococcus* causes erysipelas
- ☐ **C** Impetigo is associated with glomerulonephritis
- ☐ **D** None of the options
- ☐ **E** Scalded skin syndrome is caused by *Staphylococcus aureus*

2.40 **A leukaemic patient on chemotherapy presents with fever and a pulmonary infiltrate. Which one of the following infectious agents could present in this way?**

- ☐ **A** All of the options
- ☐ **B** *Chlamydia*
- ☐ **C** *Cryptococcus*
- ☐ **D** Herpes simplex
- ☐ **E** None of the options

2.41 **A 26-year-old man with a history of injecting drugs is admitted with fever and malaise. His temperature is 39.3 °C, pulse 126 bpm and blood pressure 90/65 mmHg. He is mildly confused, but without symptoms of meningism or focal neurological signs. A loud murmur that increases with inspiration is audible at the lower left sternal edge. A plain chest X-ray shows several small cavitating lesions peripherally, but is otherwise normal. Which one of the following is the most likely diagnosis?**

- ☐ **A** Acute HIV seroconversion illness
- ☐ **B** *Cryptococcus neoformans* infection
- ☐ **C** Mycobacterium tuberculosis infection
- ☐ **D** *Staphylococcus aureus* endocarditis and septicaemia
- ☐ **E** Tricuspid endocarditis due to *Streptococcus bovis*

2.42 **Antibiotic chemotherapies employ several mechanisms of action. Some interfere with bacterial cell-wall synthesis and others penetrate well into cells and disrupt bacterial ribosomal function. Which one of the following drugs acts by interfering with ribosomal function?**

☐ **A** Amoxicillin

☐ **B** Ciprofloxacin

☐ **C** Clarithromycin

☐ **D** Trimethoprim

☐ **E** Vancomycin

2.43 **An 85-year-old White woman presents with fever, headache, neck stiffness and photophobia. She recently completed a three-day course of cefalexin for a urinary tract infection. Her past medical history is otherwise unremarkable. A lumbar puncture is performed and the cerebrospinal fluid (CSF) is found to be clear and colourless. The CSF biochemistry and microscopy shows a protein of 1.7 g/l, a glucose of 3.1 mmol/l (plasma glucose 6.8 mmol/l), and a white cell count of 104 per mm3 (lymphocytes 65%, polymorphs 35%). Occasional short Gram-positive rods are present. Which one of the following is the likely cause of her meningitis?**

☐ **A** *Listeria monocytogenes*

☐ **B** *Mycobacterium tuberculosis*

☐ **C** *Neisseria meningitides*

☐ **D** *Pseudomonas aeruginosa*

☐ **E** *Streptococcus pneumoniae*

2.44 **Cytomegalovirus (CMV) is an important opportunistic infection in immunocompromised individuals. Of the five clinical complications of HIV infection listed below, which one would be least likely to be due to CMV infection?**

☐ **A** Acalculous cholecystitis

☐ **B** Encephalitis

☐ **C** Nephritis

☐ **D** Polyradiculopathy

☐ **E** Retinitis

Answers on pages 105–118

2.45 Which one of the following is a chemokine co-receptor that acts in conjunction with the CD4 receptor to enable attachment of the HIV virus, membrane fusion, and internalisation of the contents of the HIV virus into the host cytoplasm?

☐ **A** CCR5

☐ **B** CD8

☐ **C** gp120

☐ **D** HIV protease enzyme

☐ **E** *Pol* gene product

2.46 A 35-year-old man presents with a two-day history of fever, malaise, wheeze, mild diarrhoea, an urticarial rash and hepatosplenomegaly. He recently returned from a three-month overland trip in East Africa. He can recall numerous insect bites on his trip and his adherence to antimalarial prophylaxis has been poor. He swam in freshwater rivers and consumed local food and beverages. His full blood count on admission shows a normal haemoglobin and platelet count, but a raised white cell count of 15.7×10^9/l (neutrophils 26%, lymphocytes 21%, eosinophils 45%, monocytes 1%). No malaria parasites are detected on three separate films. Which one of the following is the most likely diagnosis?

☐ **A** Amoebiasis

☐ **B** Dengue fever

☐ **C** Leishmaniasis

☐ **D** Malaria

☐ **E** Schistosomiasis

2.47 A 43-year-old man, HIV positive for 10 years, stopped antiretroviral treatments six months ago because of side-effects. His current CD4 count is very low. Over the course of two months he has developed a hemiparesis and dysarthria, but has not been systemically unwell or febrile. A magnetic resonance imaging (MRI) scan of the brain shows multiple cerebral white matter lesions that do not enhance with contrast or show mass effect. Cerebrospinal fluid examination is within normal limits. Which one of the following organisms is most likely to be responsible for his symptoms?

☐ **A** *Cryptococcus neoformans*

☐ **B** JC virus

☐ **C** *Mycobacterium tuberculosis*

☐ **D** *Nocardia asteroides*

☐ **E** *Toxoplasma gondii*

2.48 A 25-year-old woman is admitted to hospital acutely unwell with malaise, fever, profuse vomiting, and mild diarrhoea over a 36-hour period. There is no history of foreign travel and her food history is unremarkable. On admission her pulse is 130 bpm, blood pressure 84/62 mmHg, temperature 38.9 °C. She is confused, but has no focal neurology. She has a faint, erythaematous rash, particularly noticeable on her extremities. Her tongue and buccal mucosa are noted to be red and hyperaemic. What is the most likely diagnosis?

☐ **A** *Escherichia coli* O157 infection

☐ **B** Meningococcal septicaemia

☐ **C** *Salmonella* gastroenteritis

☐ **D** Toxic shock syndrome

☐ **E** Typhoid fever

Answers on pages 105–118

2.49 A 25-year-old man presents to a sexually transmitted diseases (STD) clinic. He moved to the UK from West Africa four years ago. Five days ago he developed a cluster of ten small (1–2-mm), painful, punched-out ulcers on the penis. The inguinal lymph nodes are tender and slightly enlarged, but there is no evidence of suppuration. He has had unprotected sex with a new partner recently. Which one of the following is the most likely diagnosis?

- ☐ **A** Behçet disease
- ☐ **B** Chancroid
- ☐ **C** Genital herpes
- ☐ **D** Lymphogranuloma venereum (LGV)
- ☐ **E** Syphilis

2.50 Which one of the following statements regarding antituberculous medication is incorrect?

- ☐ **A** Capreomycin is ototoxic
- ☐ **B** Macrolides may increase the risk of rifabutin-induced uveitis
- ☐ **C** Rifampicin causes an orange discoloration of the urine and secretions
- ☐ **D** Rifampicin is a potent liver enzyme inducer
- ☐ **E** Toxic side-effects of isoniazid are best reduced by the concomitant use of rifabutin

Neurology

Best of Five

Questions

NEUROLOGY 'BEST OF FIVE' QUESTIONS

For each of the questions select the ONE most appropriate answer from the options provided.

3.1 A 42-year old man has a 2-week history of pain in the upper forearm and difficulty turning his front door key in its lock. He is unable to flex the interphalangeal joint of the thumb and has weakness of forearm pronation. What is the most likely nerve to have been damaged?

☐ **A** Anterior interosseous nerve

☐ **B** Median nerve

☐ **C** Ulnar nerve

☐ **D** Radial nerve

☐ **E** Posterior interosseous nerve

3.2 Which one of the following findings on lumbar puncture is most consistent with a diagnosis of Guillain–Barré syndrome?

☐ **A** Normal cerebrospinal fluid (CSF) protein

☐ **B** Elevated CSF leucocyte count

☐ **C** Elevated CSF glucose

☐ **D** Reduced CSF protein

☐ **E** Elevated CSF protein

3.3 Which one of the following side-effects is most likely to be caused by sodium valproate therapy?

☐ **A** Visual field defects

☐ **B** Hirsutism

☐ **C** Tremor

☐ **D** Weight loss

☐ **E** Anxiety

3.4 **Which one of the following cognitive problems is most likely to result from a frontal lobe infarction?**

☐ **A** Hemianopia

☐ **B** Visual neglect

☐ **C** Episodic memory loss

☐ **D** Perseveration

☐ **E** Acalculia

3.5 **A 21-year old college student complains of general fatigue and diplopia while reading. He has a mild right ptosis but neurological examination is otherwise normal. What is the most appropriate test to reveal the diagnosis?**

☐ **A** Muscle biopsy

☐ **B** Lumbar puncture

☐ **C** Serum anti-Hu antibodies

☐ **D** Tensilon test

☐ **E** Vital capacity measurement

3.6 **A 43-year old woman complains of acute loss of vision in one eye and pain on eye movement. What is the most likely diagnosis?**

☐ **A** Optic neuritis

☐ **B** Leber's optic neuropathy

☐ **C** Ischaemic optic neuropathy

☐ **D** Myasthenia gravis

☐ **E** Guillain–Barré syndrome

3.7 **A patient has global wasting of the small muscles of the hand. Which nerve root is most likely to be affected?**

☐ **A** C4

☐ **B** C6

☐ **C** C2

☐ **D** C8

☐ **E** T1

Answers on pages 121–133

3.8 **Which pituitary hormone is in constant inhibition?**

☐ **A** TSH

☐ **B** Prolactin

☐ **C** FSH

☐ **D** LH

☐ **E** ACTH

3.9 **Which one of the following electrophysiological findings is most consistent with a diagnosis of motor neurone disease?**

☐ **A** Normal amplitude compound muscle potential

☐ **B** Reduced amplitude sensory action potentials

☐ **C** Presence of motor conduction block

☐ **D** Fibrillation and fasciculation potentials

☐ **E** Complex repetitive dischargers

3.10 **Which one of the following blood test results is most consistent with a diagnosis of dermatomyositis?**

☐ **A** Elevated serum creatine kinase

☐ **B** Decreased serum aldolase

☐ **C** Elevated serum AST

☐ **D** Elevated serum troponin

☐ **E** Decreased serum LHD

3.11 **An obese 45-year-old woman presents with headaches and visual loss and is found to have papilloedema. A computed tomography (CT) head scan is normal. What is the most likely diagnosis?**

☐ **A** Optic neuritis

☐ **B** Benign intracranial hypertension

☐ **C** Migraine

☐ **D** Normal-pressure hydrocephalus

☐ **E** Acromegaly

3.12 A 56-year-old man presents with altered sensation in the right little finger and lateral aspect of the palm. There is weakness of the small muscles of the hand. Which nerve is most likely to be damaged?

☐ **A** Median nerve

☐ **B** Anterior interosseous nerve

☐ **C** Radial nerve

☐ **D** Ulnar nerve

☐ **E** Axillary nerve

3.13 A 22-year-old woman has a 2-day history of frontal headache and blurring of vision in the right eye, aggravated by eye movement. Her visual acuities are 6/18 (right) and 6/5 (left) with a right afferent pupillary defect. What is the most likely appearance of the optic disc in the right eye?

☐ **A** Haemorrhagic

☐ **B** Large cup

☐ **C** Swollen

☐ **D** Pale

☐ **E** Normal

3.14 A 33-year-old man presents with a sudden-onset, severe occipital headache; there are no abnormal clinical signs and computed tomography (CT) (head) is normal. What is the most important investigation to perform urgently?

☐ **A** Magnetic resonance imaging (MRI) of the brain

☐ **B** Electroencephalogram (EEG)

☐ **C** Lumbar puncture

☐ **D** Serum creatine kinase estimation

☐ **E** Electrocardiogram (ECG)

Answers on pages 121–133

3.15 A 58-year-old man presents with progressive memory loss over 2 years, occasional incontinence of urine and a shuffling gait. What is a computed tomography (CT) scan of the brain most likely to show?

☐ **A** Multiple white matter lesions

☐ **B** Parasagittal meningioma

☐ **C** Temporal lobe glioma

☐ **D** Communicating hydrocephalus

☐ **E** Normal appearance

3.16 A 63-year-old man is found to have a left homonymous hemianopia. What structure is likely to be damaged?

☐ **A** Left occipital lobe

☐ **B** Right occipital lobe

☐ **C** Left lateral geniculate nucleus

☐ **D** Optic chiasm

☐ **E** Left optic nerve

3.17 A 23-year-old man presents with the rapid onset of right leg weakness. There is decreased proprioception in the right leg and absent sensation to pinprick in the left leg. What is the most likely diagnosis?

☐ **A** Guillain–Barré syndrome

☐ **B** Intramedullary spinal cord glioma

☐ **C** Brown-Séquard syndrome

☐ **D** Anterior spinal artery occlusion

☐ **E** Lumbosacral disc herniation

3.18 A 56-year-old diabetic presents with horizontal diplopia, worse on looking to the right. The outer image disappears when the right eye is covered. Which nerve is most likely to have been affected?

☐ **A** Right oculomotor

☐ **B** Left abducens

☐ **C** Right abducens

☐ **D** Left trochlear

☐ **E** Right trochlear

3.19 A new diagnostic test for variant Creutzfeldt–Jakob disease (vCJD) has recently been published. What term describes the proportion of patients with confirmed vCJD that will be identified by the test?

☐ **A** Accuracy

☐ **B** Negative predictive value

☐ **C** Positive predictive value

☐ **D** Sensitivity

☐ **E** Specificity

3.20 A 67-year-old woman has repeated stabbing pain in the right cheek, precipitated by chewing or washing her face. What is the best initial treatment for her condition?

☐ **A** Carbamazepine

☐ **B** Propranolol

☐ **C** Benzhexol

☐ **D** Botulinum toxin

☐ **E** Methotrexate

3.21 A 67-year-old man presents with sudden onset of unsteadiness, dizziness and weakness. He has a right Horner syndrome, right-sided pyramidal weakness and loss of pinprick sensation on his left side. What is the most likely diagnosis?

☐ **A** Posterior communicating artery aneurysm

☐ **B** Occipital haemorrhage

☐ **C** Posterior inferior cerebellar artery occlusion

☐ **D** Pontine haemorrhage

☐ **E** Carotid arterial dissection

Answers on pages 121–133

3.22   A 23-year-old man has been having continuous grand mal seizures for 15 minutes, having been given lorazepam 4 mg intravenously five minutes ago. What is the most appropriate immediate treatment?

☐ **A** Intravenous diazepam 10 mg

☐ **B** Intravenous lorazepam 2 mg

☐ **C** Intravenous phenytoin 15 mg/kg

☐ **D** Oral phenytoin 300 mg

☐ **E** Intravenous phenobarbital (phenobarbital) 1 mg/kg

3.23   A 58-year-old man has memory loss that has progressed rapidly over three months. He is profoundly ataxic. What is the most likely diagnosis?

☐ **A** Pick disease

☐ **B** Creutzfeldt–Jakob disease (CJD)

☐ **C** Lewy body dementia

☐ **D** Wilson disease

☐ **E** Corticobasal dementia

3.24   A 23-year-old woman suffers a single unprovoked seizure. What advice is most appropriate to give her regarding driving a private motor vehicle?

☐ **A** No driving only if there is a further seizure

☐ **B** No driving only if a structural lesion is confirmed

☐ **C** No driving only if there are electroencephalogram (EEG) abnormalities

☐ **D** No driving for 3 years

☐ **E** No driving for 1 year

3.25   A 38-year-old man with migraine takes sumatriptan but is finding that the frequency of his migraines has increased recently to six to eight per month. What is the most appropriate medication to consider adding?

☐ **A** Haloperidol

☐ **B** Rizatriptan

☐ **C** Aspirin

☐ **D** Carbamazepine

☐ **E** Propranolol

Answers on pages 121–133

3.26   A 54-year-old woman with ovarian carcinoma develops profound ataxia. MRI (brain) is normal. What blood test is most likely to aid in making a diagnosis?

☐ **A** Anti-Hu antibodies

☐ **B** Anti-Ro antibodies

☐ **C** Anti-Yo antibodies

☐ **D** Acetylcholine receptor antibodies

☐ **E** Calcium-channel antibodies

3.27   A 32-year-old man presents with a 2-week history of gradually worsening vision in his right eye, associated with discomfort on left eye movements. Visual acuity is decreased in the right eye with a right afferent pupillary defect; fundi are normal. What is the most likely diagnosis?

☐ **A** Orbital meningioma

☐ **B** Pituitary tumour

☐ **C** Tobacco amblyopia

☐ **D** Optic neuritis

☐ **E** Ischaemic optic neuropathy

3.28   A 37-year-old HIV-positive man complains of mild right-sided weakness for 2 weeks. Computed tomography (CT) (head) shows a hypodense lesion with ring enhancement in the left basal ganglia and frontal region. What is the most likely diagnosis?

☐ **A** Cerebral vasculitis

☐ **B** Neurocysticercosis

☐ **C** Toxoplasmosis

☐ **D** Neurosyphilis

☐ **E** Cytomegalovirus encephalitis

Answers on pages 121–133

3.29 A 23-year-old woman presents with two episodes of non-sustained jerking of the left arm lasting a few minutes without loss of consciousness. MRI (brain) is normal. What is the most appropriate medication to commence?

☐ **A** Phenytoin

☐ **B** Levetiracetam

☐ **C** Carbamazepine

☐ **D** Lorazepam

☐ **E** Vigabatrin

3.30 A 48-year-old woman has recently taken antibiotics for sinusitis but develops vomiting and headache. Cerebrospinal fluid (CSF) examination demonstrates 40 white cells (80% lymphocytes), protein 0.6 g/l (normal range 0.15–0.45 g/l), normal glucose and negative Gram stain. What is the most likely diagnosis?

☐ **A** Viral meningitis

☐ **B** Partially treated bacterial meningitis

☐ **C** Cryptococcal meningitis

☐ **D** Cerebral toxoplasmosis

☐ **E** Viral encephalitis

3.31 A 75-year-old man presents with an 18-month history of progressive difficulty using his right arm, slurred speech, difficulty walking and feeling dizzy on standing. He has a resting tremor of his right arm, dysarthria and mild postural hypotension. What is the most likely diagnosis?

☐ **A** Shy–Drager syndrome

☐ **B** Idiopathic Parkinson's disease

☐ **C** Steele–Richardson–Olszewski syndrome

☐ **D** Progressive supranuclear palsy

☐ **E** Wilson disease

3.32 A 43-year-old woman complains of unsteadiness, syncope, constipation and urinary retention. She was previously well, takes no medications and has no relevant family history. On physical examination, you find bradykinesia, mild resting tremor and severe postural hypotension. Which one of the following is the most likely diagnosis?

☐ **A** Huntington disease

☐ **B** Idiopathic Parkinson disease

☐ **C** Multiple system atrophy

☐ **D** Normal-pressure hydrocephalus

☐ **E** Progressive supranuclear palsy

3.33 A 56-year-old man with poorly controlled diabetes complains of horizontal diplopia. You notice a subtle convergent strabismus. His diplopia is worse on looking to the right and, on covering his right eye, he tells you that the outer image disappears. Which one of the following cranial nerves is the most likely site of the underlying lesion?

☐ **A** Left abducens nerve

☐ **B** Left oculomotor nerve

☐ **C** Right abducens nerve

☐ **D** Right oculomotor nerve

☐ **E** Right trochlear nerve

3.34 A 58-year-old woman is brought to the Emergency Department unresponsive after collapsing at her home. Her husband reports that she felt well that morning, but developed a progressively severe headache. She has a history of hypertension and atrial fibrillation for which she is anticoagulated. On examination she has a blood pressure of 220/140 mmHg and has apnoea alternating with hyperpnoea. She responds only to noxious stimuli, with right-sided extensor posturing. She has papilloedema and an unreactive pupil on the left, diffuse hyper-reflexia and bilateral upgoing plantars. Which one of the following herniation syndromes is most consistent with her clinical presentation?

☐ **A** Brainstem through the tentorial notch

☐ **B** Cerebellar tonsils through the foramen magnum

☐ **C** Cingulate gyrus beneath the falx

☐ **D** Diencephalon through the tentorial notch

☐ **E** Temporal lobe uncus across the tentorium

Answers on pages 121–133

3.35   A 62-year-old man develops left-sided limb ataxia, left Horner syndrome, nystagmus and loss of pain and temperature sensation on the right side of his face. Which artery is most likely to be occluded?

☐ **A** Basilar artery

☐ **B** Posterior cerebral artery

☐ **C** Posterior inferior cerebellar artery

☐ **D** Superior cerebellar artery

☐ **E** Vertebral artery

3.36   A 31-year-old man gives a 3-year history of increasing deafness and tinnitus in his right ear. He is a smoker and has no other medical history. On examination, his auditory acuity is grossly impaired on the left. Rinne's test shows air conduction to be greater than bone conduction. You notice no nystagmus and balance is normal, but the left corneal reflex is absent. Which one of the following is the most likely diagnosis?

☐ **A** Acoustic neuroma

☐ **B** Basilar artery aneurysm

☐ **C** Brainstem astrocytoma

☐ **D** Multiple sclerosis

☐ **E** Nasopharyngeal carcinoma

3.37   A 52-year-old woman presents with a 3-month history of right-sided tingling, numbness and weakness. Her entire right side is completely numb, yet hypersensitive to touch. Five years earlier she underwent mastectomy for breast carcinoma. You find a hemiplegic gait, right hemianaesthesia to all sensory modalities, minimal weakness and flexor plantars. Which one of the following is most likely to be causing these symptoms and signs?

☐ **A** Left posterior cerebral artery infarction

☐ **B** Left postcentral gyrus metastasis

☐ **C** Left thalamic metastasis

☐ **D** Multiple sclerosis

☐ **E** Right cerebellar infarction

3.38   A 26-year-old man, previously healthy, complains of progressive visual loss accompanied by intermittent central headaches. On examination you note a bitemporal inferior quadrantanopia, but no other neurological abnormalities. Which one of the following diagnoses is most likely?

☐ **A** Craniopharyngioma

☐ **B** Cushing disease

☐ **C** Optic neuritis

☐ **D** Prolactinoma

☐ **E** Retinitis pigmentosa

3.39   A 48-year-old hypertensive man tripped while playing football and awoke the next day with severe foot drop. On examination, foot eversion is impaired and there is there is severe weakness of dorsiflexion. The ankle reflex is intact and there is no evidence of sensory loss. Which one of the following structures is most likely to be damaged?

☐ **A** Common peroneal nerve

☐ **B** Femoral nerve

☐ **C** L5/S1 nerve root

☐ **D** Sciatic nerve

☐ **E** Tibial nerve

3.40   A 36-year-old Asian man presents with a 2-day history of sore throat, headache and vomiting. Two years previously he underwent splenectomy following a road traffic accident. On examination, he is confused, disoriented, febrile and photophobic. He is tachycardic and you notice a petechial rash on his upper arms, together with mild neck stiffness and a positive Kernig's sign. There is no papilloedema. Which one of the following is the diagnosis?

☐ **A** *Haemophilus* meningitis

☐ **B** Herpes simplex encephalitis

☐ **C** Meningococcal meningitis

☐ **D** Pneumococcal meningitis

☐ **E** Tuberculous meningitis

Answers on pages 121–133

3.41 **A 76-year-old woman is brought to the clinic by her daughter. She is worried about her mother's increasing forgetfulness. Her mother has had increasing difficulty managing at home over several months, forgetting what she has bought and getting lost while out at the shops. The presence of which one of the following abnormalities lends most weight to a diagnosis of Alzheimer's disease?**

☐ **A** Constructional apraxia

☐ **B** Disinhibition

☐ **C** Disorientation in time

☐ **D** Episodic memory deficit

☐ **E** Visual hallucinations

3.42 **A 32-year-old woman presents with choreiform movements and intellectual decline over a period of several years. She denies any family history of neurological disorder. On examination she has continual choreiform jerks involving the hands and feet; sensation, power and reflexes are normal, with flexor plantars. Which one of the following is the most likely diagnosis?**

☐ **A** Huntington disease

☐ **B** Multiple sclerosis

☐ **C** Neuroacanthocytosis

☐ **D** Parkinson disease

☐ **E** Wilson disease

3.43 **A 68-year-old female smoker complains of progressive difficulty with writing and simple mental arithmetic. On examination you find a lower right homonymous quadrantanopia; neuropsychological testing confirms a mild dyscalculia, dysgraphia and finger agnosia. You order an MRI scan; damage to which one of the following structures do you suspect is responsible for her symptoms?**

☐ **A** Left frontal lobe

☐ **B** Left occipital lobe

☐ **C** Left parietal lobe

☐ **D** Right parietal lobe

☐ **E** Left temporal lobe

3.44 A 34-year-old woman presents complaining of episodic leg weakness and crampy abdominal pain without diarrhoea. During an episode, her abdomen is distended with decreased bowel sounds and she has distal leg weakness with loss of knee and ankle jerks. These findings suggest a defect in the biosynthetic pathway for:

- ☐ **A** Collagen
- ☐ **B** Corticosteroids
- ☐ **C** Glucose
- ☐ **D** Haem
- ☐ **E** Thyroxine

3.45 A 24-year-old man presents with a 7-day history of progressive lower limb paraesthesiae, numbness extending from both feet up to the lower abdomen and difficulty walking. Numbness has started to develop in his hands. You find generalised weakness and areflexia on examination, but without definite sensory loss. Which one of the following is the most likely diagnosis?

- ☐ **A** Cervical cord compression
- ☐ **B** Guillain–Barré syndrome
- ☐ **C** Motor neurone disease
- ☐ **D** Myasthenia gravis
- ☐ **E** Polymyositis

3.46 A 26-year-old woman presents with two episodes of loss of consciousness. On each occasion she remembers a strong smell immediately before losing consciousness. Her work colleagues who observed these episodes report that she sat motionless at her desk, chewing repetitively for a few seconds, before slumping forwards. She was unconscious for about 30 seconds, subsequently appearing confused and disoriented for a few minutes. Physical examination, electroencephalogram (EEG) and MRI are all normal. Which one of the following treatments is likely to be most appropriate?

- ☐ **A** Carbamazepine
- ☐ **B** Ethosuximide
- ☐ **C** Gabapentin
- ☐ **D** Lamotrigine
- ☐ **E** Phenytoin

 Answers on pages 121–133

3.47 A 26-year-old woman is brought to the Emergency Department having collapsed in a nightclub with a tonic–clonic seizure. When you see her, she is awake and complaining of nausea and headache. On examination she has moderate pyramidal weakness of the right leg. A computed tomography (CT) scan shows bilateral haemorrhagic infarction of the white matter in the left parietal lobe. The most likely cause is occlusion of which one of the following blood vessels?

☐ **A** Cavernous sinus

☐ **B** Left middle cerebral artery

☐ **C** Left posterior cerebral artery

☐ **D** Right anterior cerebral artery

☐ **E** Sagittal sinus

3.48 A 34-year-old vegan presents with a 6-week history of distressing paraesthesiae in the hands and legs. In the last 2 weeks, her gait has become unsteady and she feels her legs have become weak. On examination, vibration and joint-position sense is impaired in the lower limbs. Her legs show increased tone, a mild symmetrical proximal loss of power, hyper-reflexia and bilateral upgoing plantars. Her gait is ataxic. What nutritional deficiency is the likely cause of her problems?

☐ **A** Folic acid

☐ **B** Iron

☐ **C** Pyridoxine

☐ **D** Thiamine

☐ **E** Vitamin B_{12}

3.49 A 29-year-old man presents with acute onset of wrist drop 6 weeks after breaking his leg. You find weakness of forearm extension, wrist and finger extension and loss of the triceps and brachioradialis reflexes, but with little sensory loss. Which one of the following branches of the brachial plexus is most likely to be affected?

☐ **A** Axillary

☐ **B** Dorsal scapular

☐ **C** Median

☐ **D** Radial

☐ **E** Ulnar

3.50 A 52-year-old man has been suffering from progressive forgetfulness and unsteadiness of gait for 2 months. You observe spontaneous myoclonic twitching of his fingers and elicit startle myoclonus to a loud noise. Neuropsychological examination reveals profound impairment of memory, attention and language function. Which one of the following is the most likely underlying diagnosis?

- ☐ **A** Alzheimer's disease
- ☐ **B** Creutzfeldt–Jakob disease
- ☐ **C** Myoclonic epilepsy
- ☐ **D** Pick disease
- ☐ **E** Subacute sclerosing panencephalitis

Answers on pages 121–133

Psychiatry

Best of Five

Questions

PSYCHIATRY 'BEST OF FIVE' QUESTIONS

For each of the questions select the ONE most appropriate answer from the options provided.

4.1   A 30-year-old nurse has been referred to the clinic following a recent diagnosis of systemic lupus erythematosus (SLE). She feels she is having a 'nervous breakdown' and wishes to find out whether her SLE is affecting her mind. She is asking for advice on this matter. Which one of the following statements is most likely with regard to SLE and mental disorder?

☐ **A**   Cerebral manifestations occur in less than 10% of cases

☐ **B**   Schizophreniform psychosis is the commonest psychiatric manifestation

☐ **C**   Psychiatric symptoms are usually due to cerebral arteritis

☐ **D**   Psychiatric symptoms usually precede fever and arthralgia

☐ **E**   Cerebral involvement is an indicator of poor prognosis

4.2   A 56-year-old man has been admitted following an episode of chest pain. He has a history of schizophrenia and has been on a depot antipsychotic for a number of years. You notice that he has quite marked abnormal involuntary movements. Movements include choreoathetosis and orofacial dyskinesia and you conclude he has tardive dyskinesia (TD). Which one of the following statements regarding tardive dyskinesia is most accurate?

☐ **A**   It is associated with previous brain damage

☐ **B**   It occurs in most patients on long-term neuroleptic treatment

☐ **C**   It is more common in men

☐ **D**   It is associated with reduced life expectancy in severe schizophrenia

☐ **E**   It invariably improves on stopping the offending neuroleptic

4.3 A 28-year-old woman has recently given birth to her first child. She presents to the Emergency Department complaining that the child is severely ill as he never stops crying. The child has been examined and does not appear to be unwell. However, you are concerned that the mother is exhibiting signs of mental disorder and may be in need of treatment. Which one of the following characteristics would most support a diagnosis of puerperal psychosis?

☐ **A** Onset of symptoms within 2 days of the birth

☐ **B** Onset of symptoms after 2 weeks from the birth

☐ **C** Clouding of consciousness

☐ **D** A past history of schizophrenia

☐ **E** Despondency as the predominant underlying affective state

4.4 You see a patient in the neurology clinic who is complaining of short-term memory loss. Which of the following features of his examination make it most likely he is not suffering from dementia?

☐ **A** Says he does not know the answers and cannot do the tests

☐ **B** Low mood

☐ **C** Personality changes

☐ **D** Problems with short-term memory

☐ **E** Family history of depression

4.5 A 47-year-old woman has been admitted to the ward in a severely dehydrated state. The history obtained from her husband is that his wife has been very depressed following the death of their only child. Over the past few weeks she has hardly been eating and is now refusing any fluids. An emergency course of electroconvulsive therapy (ECT) has been prescribed by the psychiatrists, under the provisions of the Mental Health Act. The husband is concerned about the ECT and asks you a number of questions regarding the treatment. Which one of his concerns regarding the proposed ECT is most valid?

☐ **A** ECT can cause permanent damage to memory

☐ **B** ECT can cause short-term memory loss

☐ **C** Patients appear distressed during ECT, with arms and legs convulsing

☐ **D** There is no good quality evidence demonstrating efficacy of ECT

☐ **E** An antidepressant would be as effective as ECT for his wife and should be used in preference

Answers on pages 137–148

4.6   **A 48-year-old man frequently attends the clinic claiming that there has been no improvement in his symptoms despite several appropriate interventions. He does appear unhappy and you query whether he might be depressed. Which one of his following symptoms would most suggest a course of an antidepressant might lead to some improvement?**

☐   **A**   Incongruity of mood and thinking

☐   **B**   Episodes of irritability and increased tempo of thought

☐   **C**   Improvement of mood every evening

☐   **D**   Chronic anhedonia

☐   **E**   Fluctuating levels of concentration

4.7   **A 30-year-old woman presents with an exacerbation of long-standing asthma. She describes intermittent attacks of dyspnoea accompanied by prominent palpitations and tremor. She describes being very anxious during an attack and you query whether she has coexisting panic disorder that would benefit from treatment. The presence of which one of the following symptoms would add weight to the diagnosis of panic disorder?**

☐   **A**   There is usually a clear precipitant to the attack

☐   **B**   There is an accompanying sense of impending doom

☐   **C**   Attacks last approximately 1 hour

☐   **D**   Staying as still as possible in one place helps the attack to subside

☐   **E**   The patient has underlying near-continuous feelings of nervousness in between attacks

4.8   **You are asked to see a 40-year-old man on a surgical ward who is complaining of atypical chest pain. He had an abdominal operation five days ago. The surgeons report clouding of consciousness for the first day postoperation but none since. After assessing the patient you still suspect the patient may have an acute confusional state (delirium). Which one of the following features would be most consistent with this diagnosis?**

☐   **A**   Abnormal psychomotor activity

☐   **B**   Autotopagnosia

☐   **C**   Catastrophic reaction

☐   **D**   Thought alienation

☐   **E**   Labile affect

Questions: Psychiatry

4.9 A patient is admitted suffering from recurrent falls. His wife reports he has also had some memory problems. He fluctuates on a day to day basis and can be variable in his ability. Which one of the following findings makes a diagnosis of Lewy body dementia most likely?

- ☐ **A** Sensitivity to neuroleptics
- ☐ **B** Postural hypotension
- ☐ **C** Confusing dreams with reality
- ☐ **D** Depression
- ☐ **E** Visual hallucinations

4.10 A 65-year-old man was admitted after being found unconscious on the street smelling of alcohol. He was initially confused and had been on the ward for 2 weeks when his behaviour changed. He became agitated and talkative. He developed short-term memory problems and got lost on the ward, forgetting where the bathroom is. He has persistent beliefs that he spends all day at work and that the ward is a hotel that he returns to in the evening. An occupational therapy assessment shows no impairment of daily living skills. What is the most likely diagnosis?

- ☐ **A** Schizophrenia
- ☐ **B** Delirium
- ☐ **C** Korsakoff syndrome
- ☐ **D** Alzheimer disease
- ☐ **E** Alcoholic hallucinosis

4.11 You are asked to see a 35-year-old woman on a surgical ward who had a gastric banding procedure for morbid obesity 6 months ago. Her digit span is impaired and she is disorientated in time and place. Which one of the following symptoms most supports a diagnosis of Wernicke syndrome?

- ☐ **A** Anterograde amnesia
- ☐ **B** Hyperintense lesions on MRI imaging of the medial thalamus
- ☐ **C** Ataxia
- ☐ **D** Nystagmus
- ☐ **E** Peripheral neuropathy

Answers on pages 137–148

4.12 A 15-year-old post-pubertal girl has been admitted in an emaciated state. She says she has lost her appetite because of the stress of taking examinations. She strongly denies being anorexic. Which one of the following from your assessment of her would lend most weight to a diagnosis of anorexia nervosa?

☐ **A** A body mass index (BMI) of 16.5 kg/m^2

☐ **B** A denial that she is underweight

☐ **C** A previous history of bulimia nervosa

☐ **D** Amenorrhoea

☐ **E** Episodes of intermittent binge eating when unobserved

4.13 A 28-year-old man has been admitted having collapsed in the street. He refuses to speak to you. You suspect from his behaviour that he has a mental illness, but the patient denies this and you cannot access his GP out of hours. The only information you have is a list of his prescribed medication found by ambulance staff. In trying to distinguish which mental illness he may have, which one of the following of his medications would be least likely to be prescribed for a patient with schizoaffective disorder?

☐ **A** Chlordiazepoxide

☐ **B** Clozapine

☐ **C** Haloperidol

☐ **D** Procyclidine

☐ **E** Sodium valproate

Questions: Psychiatry

4.14 You are reviewing a 46-year-old woman with multiple sclerosis in the clinic. Since starting on fluoxetine (a selective serotonin re-uptake inhibitor, SSRI) 4 months ago, her quality of life has improved and she no longer presents as feeling hopeless about the future. However, she states her antidepressant has given her a number of side-effects and she wishes to stop taking it. You attempt to reassure her that most of her symptoms are unlikely to be attributable to fluoxetine, except for which one of the following?

☐ **A** Anorgasmia

☐ **B** Extrapyramidal side-effects

☐ **C** Sedation

☐ **D** Suicidal thoughts

☐ **E** Withdrawal symptoms if she misses a dose

4.15 A 24-year-old man with well controlled diabetes attends for review in clinic. He appears low and when you ask him about his mood he says that most of the time he feels tired and depressed; everything is an effort and nothing is enjoyable. He sleeps badly and feels inadequate, but holds down a job and can cope with the basic demands of everyday life. The most likely diagnosis is?

☐ **A** Depressive disorder

☐ **B** Dysthymic disorder

☐ **C** Bipolar disorder

☐ **D** Cyclothymia

☐ **E** Brief depressive episode

Answers on pages 137–148

4.16. A 23-year-old woman presents to casualty complaining of 'unstable moods'. On questioning she describes short impersistent periods of mild depression and short periods of feeling energetic and very happy (which she finds enjoyable). Despite her difficulties she has never had any time off work, sleeps well with a good appetite and has never behaved in an inappropriate manner. She tells you her mother had 'manic depression'. The most likely diagnosis is:

- ☐ **A** Bipolar disorder
- ☐ **B** Depressive disorder
- ☐ **C** Dysthymia
- ☐ **D** Manic episode
- ☐ **E** Cyclothymia

4.17 A 48-year-old man has been referred for a medical opinion by his psychiatrist. The patient initially presented with treatment-resistant depression. He now presents with intellectual deterioration and abnormal involuntary movements. Having assessed him, you determine that the patient is not aware of any family history of a movement disorder. Despite this, you suspect Huntington disease and order an MRI brain scan. Which one of the following abnormalities on a brain scan would provide most evidence for Huntington disease?

- ☐ **A** Basal ganglia atrophy
- ☐ **B** Caudate atrophy
- ☐ **C** Dilated ventricles
- ☐ **D** Global atrophy
- ☐ **E** Temporal lobe atrophy

4.18 You are reviewing a 35-year-old man with Down syndrome at a yearly follow-up clinic for his cardiac problems. His carer accompanies him and states that the patient's behaviour has started to deteriorate and that he suspects a problem with his mental health. Which one of the following would be the most likely psychiatric cause?

- ☐ **A** Alzheimer dementia
- ☐ **B** Temporolimbic epilepsy
- ☐ **C** Manic depression
- ☐ **D** Panic disorder
- ☐ **E** Schizophrenia

4.19 A 56-year-old man being treated for Parkinson disease has started to develop intrusive auditory hallucinations. You suspect levodopa has contributed to the development of psychosis. Despite reducing his medication, the hallucinations persist and you decide to start an antipsychotic. In considering an appropriate treatment which will not exacerbate the patient's parkinsonian symptoms, which one of the following antipsychotics has the least effect on D_2 dopamine receptors?

- ☐ **A** Chlorpromazine
- ☐ **B** Haloperidol
- ☐ **C** Quetiapine
- ☐ **D** Risperidone
- ☐ **E** Sulpiride

4.20 A 62-year-old female patient is acting bizarrely on the ward. After assessing her you believe she is not acutely confused but is psychotic. The presence of which one of the following would provide evidence that the patient is acutely psychotic?

- ☐ **A** Autochthonous delusions
- ☐ **B** Echopraxia
- ☐ **C** Hypnagogical hallucinations
- ☐ **D** Hypnapompic hallucinations
- ☐ **E** Tardive dyskinesia

4.21 You are called to the ward as the nursing staff are concerned that a 34-year-old male patient has been standing in the ward office for an hour and is refusing to move. You find that the patient is alert but unresponsive. You attempt to examine the patient. Which one of the following motor disturbances would most lead you to suspect catatonia?

- ☐ **A** Reduced tone
- ☐ **B** Catalepsy
- ☐ **C** Cataplexy
- ☐ **D** Stereotypy
- ☐ **E** Mannerisms

Answers on pages 137–148

4.22 A 19-year-old man attends your clinic with his carer and is presenting with dyspnoea. The carer explains that the patient has learning difficulties but is unsure of the exact cause. Which one of the following would most support a diagnosis of fragile-X syndrome?

☐ **A** Absence of male secondary sexual characteristics

☐ **B** Tall stature

☐ **C** Prognathism

☐ **D** Single palmar crease

☐ **E** Strabismus

4.23 A 72-year-old man is in your clinic for routine follow up of his renal function. His wife mentions that he is becoming very forgetful and is irritable when she challenges him about this. He has become lost when driving on one occasion and she has noticed that he sometimes puts dirty clothes on. Which of the following most suggests he has a diagnosis of Alzheimer disease?

☐ **A** His 80-year-old brother also has dementia

☐ **B** He appears depressed

☐ **C** He has apraxia on bedside testing

☐ **D** Incontinence

☐ **E** Abnormal gait

4.24 A 28-year-old man has been referred following an overdose of 100 paracetamol tablets. Blood levels reveal a paracetamol level of zero. He also claims to have considerable abdominal pain but does not appear distressed and physical examination reveals no abnormalities except for a number of abdominal scars. The patient is admitted to hospital for observation. Which one of the following would add most weight to a diagnosis of Munchausen syndrome?

☐ **A** The prospect of financial gain from illness

☐ **B** The presence of alcohol dependence

☐ **C** The presence of secondary gain

☐ **D** Delusions of grandeur

☐ **E** Describing hearing unseen voices outside the patient's head

4.25 A 34-year-old man has been referred for an urgent medical opinion. He has been very agitated and has been treated with high doses of antipsychotics. The referring psychiatrist describes a number of clinical features that are suggestive of neuroleptic malignant syndrome. Which one of the following features is least compatible with this diagnosis?

- ☐ **A** Mutism
- ☐ **B** Dysphagia
- ☐ **C** Diaphoresis
- ☐ **D** Incontinence
- ☐ **E** Bradycardia

4.26 A 25-year-old woman is admitted with acute abdominal pain. She denies restricting her food intake but appears preoccupied with her weight. She admits to self-induced vomiting. On examination and investigation you are most likely to find?

- ☐ **A** Hyperkalaemia
- ☐ **B** Decreased growth hormone levels
- ☐ **C** Hypocholesterolaemia
- ☐ **D** Relative lymphopenia
- ☐ **E** Increased plasma amylase

4.27 A 30-year-old woman presents claiming her heart is failing. You find no abnormalities on physical examination but you elicit a number of abnormalities on mental state examination. The presence of which one of the following abnormalities lends most weight to a diagnosis of schizophrenia?

- ☐ **A** Catatonia
- ☐ **B** Gustatory hallucinations
- ☐ **C** Primary delusion
- ☐ **D** Neologisms
- ☐ **E** Tangential responses to questioning

Answers on pages 137–148

4.28 A 22-year-old man admitted following an overdose appears to be suspicious and uncommunicative. His mother says he has been very withdrawn and recently dropped out of his university course. Which of the following symptoms is least likely to suggest that he has developed schizophrenia?

- ☐ **A** Thought insertion
- ☐ **B** Delusional perceptions
- ☐ **C** Second person auditory hallucinations
- ☐ **D** Feelings influenced by external agents
- ☐ **E** Hallucinations in the form of a running commentary

4.29 A 57-year-old married man with chronic renal failure describes poor energy levels and disturbed sleep. He goes on to describe anhedonia, guilt and hopelessness and appears unhappy. You believe he is depressed. The patient will not consider antidepressants, but agrees to talk to a therapist. Which one of the following psychological treatments is likely to be most effective?

- ☐ **A** Cognitive behavioural therapy
- ☐ **B** Family therapy
- ☐ **C** Psychoanalysis
- ☐ **D** Psychodynamic therapy
- ☐ **E** Supportive therapy

4.30 A relative of a patient with schizophrenia asks you whether her son is likely to make a good recovery. Which of the following indicates that he may make a good recovery?

- ☐ **A** Onset at age 35
- ☐ **B** Florid affective symptoms
- ☐ **C** Long initial psychotic episode
- ☐ **D** He lacks insight
- ☐ **E** Soft neurological signs

Answers on pages 137–148

4.31   A 38-year-old colleague complains of being under considerable stress at work and fears that he is becoming mentally unwell. He describes a number of recent unusual experiences. Which one of the following would most lead you to suspect the presence of a psychotic disorder?

☐ **A**   Depersonalisation

☐ **B**   Derealisation

☐ **C**   Hypnagogical hallucinations

☐ **D**   Hypnapompic hallucinations

☐ **E**   Thought alienation

4.32   A 19-year-old man admitted 4 days ago appears to be experiencing auditory hallucinations and thought broadcasting and has expressed persecutory delusions to the nursing staff. His girlfriend admits he has experimented with a drug of abuse before admission. Which one of the following drugs is most likely to produce a schizophreniform psychosis?

☐ **A**   Amphetamine

☐ **B**   Cannabis

☐ **C**   Heroin

☐ **D**   LSD

☐ **E**   Psilocybin

4.33   You are reviewing a 56-year-old woman with angina in the clinic. She was widowed 1 month ago and you are concerned about the state of her mental health. Which one of the following would make you most concerned that this woman is demonstrating pathological grief?

☐ **A**   Inability to feel sadness

☐ **B**   Intense yearning for her dead husband

☐ **C**   Loss of appetite

☐ **D**   Poor sleep

☐ **E**   Visions of her dead husband

Answers on pages 137–148

4.34 A 30-year-old male political refugee has been attending hospital for several months complaining of abdominal pains. Despite extensive investigations, no organic cause has been identified. Further history-taking leads you to query the relevance of possible psychological factors. Which one of the following features would most support a diagnosis of post-traumatic stress disorder (PTSD)?

☐ **A** Believing his persecutors have followed him to the UK

☐ **B** Diurnal variation of mood

☐ **C** Early-morning wakening

☐ **D** Intrusive flashbacks

☐ **E** Panic attacks

4.35 A 25-year-old man of Afro-Caribbean origin is brought to casualty having 'collapsed'. He is currently a patient on a long-stay psychiatric unit. His electrocardiogram (ECG) shows a QTc interval of 500 ms. On inspection of his drug chart, which one of the following medications are most likely to have caused this?

☐ **A** Diazepam

☐ **B** Thioridazine

☐ **C** Flupenthixol

☐ **D** Risperidone

☐ **E** Chlorpromazine

4.36 A 45-year-old woman has been complaining of multiple, varying gastrointestinal symptoms for 3 years. Despite extensive investigations and second opinions, she refuses to accept that there is no physical explanation for her symptoms. She complains her life has been completely disrupted because of her symptoms and wants more tests to seek an answer. From the information given, which one of the following diagnoses is most appropriate?

☐ **A** Conversion disorder

☐ **B** Dissociative disorder

☐ **C** Hypochondriacal disorder

☐ **D** Hysterical disorder

☐ **E** Somatisation disorder

4.37 An 85-year-old man has been treated for an acute urinary tract infection. His wife says that he appears to be confused and has short-term memory loss. He also appears to have a flat affect and be tearful. A diagnosis of pseudodementia would be suggested by:

☐ **A** Acute onset

☐ **B** Abnormal EEG

☐ **C** Presence of localizing neurological signs

☐ **D** Performance on cognitive testing worsens during the day

☐ **E** Chronic course

4.38 A mother accompanies her 30-year-old son to the clinic. He has been referred for poor energy levels and fatigue. You discover that he has previously been treated for schizophrenia but no longer attends psychiatric follow-up. Assessment and investigations reveal no obvious cause for lethargy and you suspect the patient may be suffering negative symptoms of schizophrenia. Which one of the following is not a feature of negative schizophrenia?

☐ **A** Alogia

☐ **B** Anhedonia

☐ **C** Avolition

☐ **D** Blunting of affect

☐ **E** Negativism

4.39 A 74-year-old man has been referred to you, as over the past few weeks his behaviour has been becoming increasingly bizarre. As part of your assessment you perform a cognitive examination. Which one of the following abnormalities is most suggestive of frontal lobe dysfunction?

☐ **A** Hypersomnia

☐ **B** Impaired 5-minute recall

☐ **C** Perseverating responses

☐ **D** Right–left disorientation

☐ **E** Sensory dysphasia

Answers on pages 137–148

4.40 A 32-year-old man with no known history of mental illness presents in a highly agitated state. He appears to be experiencing distressing hallucinations and persecutory delusions. His behaviour is becoming increasingly aggressive and is no longer manageable. Which one of the following would be the most appropriate initial pharmacological intervention?

☐ **A** Intramuscular chlorpromazine

☐ **B** Intramuscular diazepam

☐ **C** Intramuscular haloperidol

☐ **D** Intramuscular lorazepam

☐ **E** Intravenous haloperidol

4.41 A 29-year-old man refuses to undress and lie on a couch for a physical examination. He states that the couch is dirty and that he does not want to risk getting an infection. Which one of the following features would most lead you to suspect a diagnosis of obsessive–compulsive disorder?

☐ **A** Acknowledging that this belief is irrational, but still refusing

☐ **B** Believing that all hospital couches are contaminated by bacteria and are an infection risk

☐ **C** Having a panic attack when approaching the couch

☐ **D** Hearing a voice telling him the couch is infected

☐ **E** Performing an elaborate, enjoyable prayer ritual before undressing

4.42 One year after a severe head injury, which one of the following cognitive deficits is most likely to be present?

☐ **A** Disorder of executive functioning

☐ **B** Fluent dysphasia

☐ **C** Non-fluent dysphasia

☐ **D** Non-verbal IQ loss

☐ **E** Short-term memory loss

4.43 A patient on long-term lithium treatment for prophylaxis of bipolar affective disorder is complaining of feeling unwell. You wish to exclude lithium toxicity as a possible diagnosis. Which one of the following abnormalities is most likely to indicate toxicity?

☐ **A** Ataxia

☐ **B** Diarrhoea

☐ **C** Metallic taste

☐ **D** Oedema

☐ **E** Tremor

4.44 A General Practitioner has finally referred a 49-year-old woman to your clinic for long-standing weakness of her left arm. The GP confirms that this symptom has been present for three years. Following your assessment, you suspect a motor conversion disorder. Which one of the following features would not lend weight to the diagnosis?

☐ **A** A state of indifference to the paralysis

☐ **B** An obvious precipitant

☐ **C** Fasciculations

☐ **D** Muscle wasting

☐ **E** Significant secondary gain

4.45 A 24-year-old woman has been brought to hospital after collapsing. She appears physically well but says she has not been eating much. You suspect an eating disorder may have contributed to her presentation and take a detailed history. Which one of the following statements would not be true of bulimia nervosa?

☐ **A** Compensatory behaviour to counteract the fattening effect of food must be present

☐ **B** There are frequent episodes of fasting

☐ **C** There are overvalued ideas of shape/weight

☐ **D** There is a loss of control over eating

☐ **E** The majority of cases are preceded by anorexia nervosa

 Answers on pages 137–148

ANSWERS

Basic Sciences

BASIC SCIENCES: 'BEST OF FIVE' ANSWERS

1.1   D: It leads to improved secretion of insulin

GLP-1 is secreted by L cells in response to the presence of nutrients in the small intestine. It leads to improvements in glucose-dependent insulin secretion and reduced production of glucagon. Weight loss may be promoted by a combination of reduced gastrointestinal (GI) motility and action on the hypothalamus. Endogenous GLP-1 is rapidly degraded and is not suitable for use as a therapeutic agent, although modification of amino acids blocks DPP-IV, the enzyme responsible for its degradation. GLP-1 analogues, which are slowly degraded, include exenatide, although this still needs to be given twice a day. Daily and weekly GLP-1 analogues are under development. Due to reduced GI motility a feeling of fullness or nausea is common among users.

1.2   B: They lead to phosphorylation of proteins

Utilising ATP as the substrate. The main purpose of receptor tyrosine kinases is to facilitate signal transduction and so up-regulate intracellular enzyme activity. As such, they play an important role in stimulating tumour growth. Sunitinib is a tyrosine kinase inhibitor that has shown activity in metastatic renal cell carcinoma and against gastric stromal tumours that have relapsed after imatinib therapy.

1.3   D: Abnormalities in cardiac sodium channels may increase the QT interval

The QT interval is associated with cardiac muscle repolarisation. Both sodium and potassium ion channel abnormalities may lead to long QT syndrome, which leads to an increased risk of ventricular arrhythmias and sudden death. Studies have now shown that the most appropriate treatment for high-risk long QT syndrome is the implantable cardioverter/defibrillator. Arrest events are usually triggered by exercise or extreme emotion.

1.4   B: Licorice excess

Natural licorice contains glycyrrhizic acid, which has both mineralocorticoid and glucocorticoid properties. Of course, the most likely explanation here is simple obesity, apart from the fact that he is hypokalaemic despite being on ramipril, a strong pointer to another underlying cause. Patients who take excess licorice for a prolonged period may present with dangerous levels of hypertension. The condition can be distinguished from Conn's in that aldosterone levels are actually low. Licorice also leads to reduced levels of testosterone and may be considered as adjunctive natural therapy for hirsutism in some patients.

1.5 C: Protein C has anti-inflammatory activity

Protein C inhibits thrombin generation through proteolysis of key co-factors involved in the clotting cascade. Protein C deficiency has equal sex incidence and heterozygous protein C deficiency usually presents around the age of 30 years, use of the oral contraceptive pill increases the risk of thrombosis. Patients with heterozygous deficiency usually have less than 60% of normal protein C activity. Homozygotes often present within a few hours after birth. A patient such as this woman would require lifelong anticoagulation.

1.6 C: It stimulates hepatic glucose output

Glucagon is a 29 amino acid polypeptide that activates glycogenolysis and gluconeogenesis. It also stimulates lipolysis and catecholamine secretion and stimulates urinary excretion of water, sodium, calcium and magnesium ions. Glucagonomas are rarely associated with MEN-1 and are associated with serum glucagon levels of more than 1000 ng/l. Necrolytic migrating erythaema, the skin rash seen here is a feature of glucagonoma in more than 80% of cases.

1.7 B: Renal bicarbonate reabsorption is increased

This man has a compensated respiratory acidosis. Chronic respiratory acidosis due to CO_2 retention is compensated for over a period of 3–5 days via increased renal carbonic acid secretion and increased renal bicarbonate reabsorption. There is also up-regulated production of NH_3 and HCO_3 by the renal brush border. Other causes of respiratory acidosis include neuromuscular diseases such as myasthenia gravis and Guillain– Barré syndrome and structural changes to the thoracic cage such as those occurring in spina bifida.

1.8 E: Autoimmune thyroid disease occurs more commonly in patients with this condition

This patient has pernicious anaemia, due to intrinsic factor autoantibodies. Vitamin B_{12} absorbtion is a complex process which begins when vitamin B_{12} becomes bound to binding proteins present in gastric juice, when this complex reaches the small intestine the binding proteins dissociate, there is binding to intrinsic factor and absorbtion via ileal receptors into the portal circulation. Oral vitamin B_{12} supplementation is ineffective, so it is given as regular intramuscular injections. Other autoimmune diseases, such as autoimmune hypothyroidism, occur more commonly in patients with pernicious anaemia.

1.9   E: The posterior area

The electrocardiogram (ECG) changes here fit with a posterior myocardial infarction. The posterior wall is usually supplied by the posterior descending coronary artery. This is supplied by the left circumflex artery in patients who have a left dominant coronary circulation, most often this area is supplied via the right coronary artery.

1.10   B: Formaldehyde accumulates in methanol toxicity

Due to alcohol dehydrogenase activity, methanol overdose leads firstly to accumulation of formaldehyde and then to formic acid. Patients develop a raised anion gap metabolic acidosis with hypotension, vomiting and acute gastrointestinal (GI) haemorrhage, death occurs at levels of methanol above around 150 mg/dl. Chronic sequelae of methanol toxicity include cataract formation, central nervous system (CNS) and hepatic dysfunction. Management of acute methanol toxicity includes competitive inhibition of alcohol dehydrogenase using ethanol or inhibition using fomepizole.

1.11   C: It occurs due to a defect in haem synthesis

This woman has acute intermittent porphyria, a condition that is commoner in women and subjects of Scandinavian or Northern European descent. It is a defect in haem synthesis, specifically in the enzyme porphobilinogen deaminase. This leads to an accumulation of porphobilinogen and amino-levulinic acid. Patients present with abdominal pain, raised blood pressure (BP) and central nervous system (CNS) symptoms, but not with the skin rash seen in other porphyrias. Oestrogens may be a potential trigger among a number of other drugs. High doses of glucose may be useful in managing mild acute attacks, with haematin infusion an option for severe patients.

1.12   D: A mutation in the *SLC5A2* gene may be the cause

This woman most probably suffers from familial renal glycosuria, which has recently been identified as due to a mutation in the *SLC5A2* gene. This codes for SGLT-2, the sodium, glucose lithium co-transporter responsible for reabsorption of glucose in the kidney back into the circulation. SGLT-1 is responsible predominantly for the absorbtion of glucose from the gastrointestinal (GI) tract. The condition is remarkably benign and is not associated with increased risk of hypertension or type-2 diabetes.

1.13   D: IL-6 is involved in the inflammatory pathway

This woman has suffered a delayed hypersensitivity reaction probably related to exposure to poison ivy. Local immune and tissue inflammatory responses at the site of exposure upregulate endothelial cell adhesion molecule expression, leading to accumulation of T-lymphocytes and macrophages, which secrete IL-1, IL-2 and IL-6. Topical corticosteroids are the mainstay of treatment, coupled with avoidance of exposure in the future.

1.14   C: Glucuronyl transferase defect is the most likely cause

This man has Gilbert syndrome, associated with a defect in UDP glucuronyl-transferase, which is commoner in men than women. It leads to transient increases in unconjugated bilirubin, which are precipitated, by acute illness or a period of fasting. Barbiturates induce the liver enzymes responsible for bilirubin processing and lead to resolution of jaundice. The condition is benign and there are no long-term sequelae.

1.15   D: They lead to profound decreases in hepatic fat

PPAR-γ agonists lead to up-regulation of a number of genes particularly associated with the handling of free fatty acids. They promote decreases in central fat stores, particularly those in the liver and differentiation of peripheral pre-adipocytes to adipocytes, which can store more lipid. This leads to a fall in insulin resistance, a decrease in lipid substrate for fuel and hence increased metabolism of circulating glucose. They promote a rise in HDL cholesterol, although they are not a primary treatment for dyslipidaemia.

1.16   C: All his offspring have a 50% chance of inheriting the disease

Huntington disease is an autosomal dominant disorder, ie it results from mutation of one copy (allele) of a gene carried on an autosome. There is full penetrance so all individuals with the genetic mutation manifest the disease. The gene affected is on chromosome 4 and produces a protein called huntingtin. Within this gene there is expansion of the CAG trinucleotide repeat. Other trinucleotide repeat disorders include: myotonic dystrophy, fragile-X syndrome, Friedreich's ataxia, spinocerebellar atrophy and spinobulbar muscular atrophy. In normal individuals the number of trinucleotide repeats varies slightly but remains below a defined threshold. Affected patients have expansion above the disease-causing threshold. The length of the expansion increases as cells divide throughout life (somatic instability) and corresponds with the age of onset of disease. The expansions enlarge further in successive generations, causing increased disease severity and earlier onset (anticipation).

Onset of Huntington chorea usually occurs in the third or fourth decade. Patients usually present with chorea (a continuous flow of jerky movements from limb to limb) and cognitive decline. There is usually a positive family history. Other presenting symptoms include dysarthria, dysphagia, ataxia, myoclonus and dystonia. Childhood onset is atypical and may be associated with rigidity. Neuropathologically, the disease causes neuronal loss in the cortex and striatum, especially in the caudate nucleus. Treatment is unsatisfactory and does not prevent progression. Neuroleptics may help reduce chorea by inhibiting dopaminergic transmission. Death usually occurs 10 to 20 years after disease onset. Genetic testing and counselling is available for patients and asymptomatic relatives.

1.17   E: When both parents carry the gene each of their offspring has a 25% chance of being affected and a 50% chance of being a carrier

Wilson disease is an autosomal recessive disorder with a gene frequency of 1 in 400 and a disease prevalence of approximately 1 in 200 000. The responsible gene is on chromosome 13 and codes for a copper-transporting ATPase. Autosomal recessive disorders result from mutations in both copies (alleles) of an autosomal gene. Both sexes are usually equally affected. Heterozygotes are carriers.

1.18   D: It allows specific DNA sequences to be amplified from a single cell

The polymerase chain reaction is an amplification reaction in which a small amount of DNA (the template) is amplified to produce enough to perform analysis. Two oligonucleotide primers are mixed with a DNA template and a thermostable DNA polymerase (*Taq* polymerase) derived from *T. aquaticus,* an organism that inhabits thermal springs. The mixture is heated to just below 100 °C and the DNA dissociates into two single strands. As the mixture cools, the oligonucleotide primers bind to either side of the specific area of interest in the DNA. The reaction is heated to 72 °C for about a minute and the DNA polymerase catalyses the synthesis of a copy of the DNA between the two primers. The process can be repeated many times to make multiple copies of the gene of interest. PCR is extremely powerful: to detect a given sequence of DNA it only needs to be present in one copy, ie one molecule of DNA. Clinical applications of PCR include:

- mutation detection
- detection of viral and bacterial sequences in tissue (eg TB, HSV, hepatitis C, HIV)

- prenatal diagnosis, from chorionic villus sampling, of known genetic mutations, eg cystic fibrosis, Duchenne muscular dystrophy
- PCR of in vitro fertilised embryo to diagnose genetic disease before implantation
- forensic medicine.

Reverse transcription PCR enables us to investigate what genes in the total genome are expressed. It does this by amplifying those genes that are being transcribed into messenger RNA (mRNA). RNA is too unstable to be used in PCR: it needs to be converted to complementary DNA (cDNA) using reverse transcriptase. This retroviral enzyme makes a precise copy of mRNA. PCR is then performed in the usual way. Because the template reflects the mRNA of the starting material, this technique can look at gene expression in individual tissues. Clinical applications of reverse transcription PCR include:

- basic scientific research into the normal function of genes by understanding their expression
- detection of the expression of particular genes in tumour tissue
- detection of RNA viruses in tissue.

Stem E describes Southern blotting, a technique used to detect and determine the size of specific restriction fragments in DNA and hence detect a specific gene of interest.

1.19   E: Paralysis of the thenar muscles, ie opponens pollicis, abductor pollicis brevis and flexor pollicis brevis

The median nerve arises from the lateral and medial cords of the brachial plexus (C6–8, T1) and sends a motor supply to:

- the lateral two lumbricals (L)
- opponens pollicis (O), abductor pollicis brevis (A) and flexor pollicis brevis (F), ie the thenar eminence muscles
- all the muscles on the flexor aspect of the forearm apart from flexor carpi ulnaris and the ulnar half of the flexor digitorum profundus.

It supplies sensation to the palmar aspect of the thumb and the lateral two and a half fingers. Median nerve damage at the wrist causes paralysis and wasting of the thenar muscles. Median nerve damage at the elbow also causes ulnar deviation and weak wrist flexion. Pronation of the forearm is lost. The signs described in stems A, B and C are features of ulnar nerve damage. Wrist drop is caused by damage to the radial nerve.

1.20   D: Temporal lobe lesion

Lesions at the optic radiation in the temporal lobe result in a contralateral homonymous hemianopia. Lesions at the optic chiasma typically produce a bitemporal hemianopia. A lesion in the right parietal lobe would result in a contralateral inferior quadrantanopia. Posterior cerebral artery occlusion tends to produce a contralateral homonymous hemianopia with macular sparing. (The macular region of the occipital cortex is on the tip of the occipital lobe, a vascular watershed area supplied by the posterior and middle cerebral arteries. Therefore it may be spared when a posterior cerebral artery CVA occurs.) Optic neuritis typically causes an ipsilateral central scotoma.

1.21   E: Metoclopramide

Galactorrhoea is caused by excess prolactin secretion. Prolactin release from the pituitary is under negative control by dopamine from the hypothalamus. Therefore dopamine and dopamine agonists, like bromocriptine, reduce prolactin release. Dopamine antagonists (such as metoclopramide) increase prolactin release. Other causes of hyperprolactinaemia and galactorrhoea are:

- pregnancy
- stress, eg epileptic fit
- oestrogens (oral contraceptive pill)
- phenothiazines (like metoclopramide, are dopamine antagonists)
- damage to the hypothalamus or pituitary stalk, eg by radiation or tumour
- renal or hepatic failure
- nipple stimulation
- polycystic ovarian syndrome.

1.22   E: Amiodarone toxicity

The patient has biochemical evidence of hepatitis and hyperthyroidism. His PFTs suggest a restrictive deficit with decreased transfer factor. In a patient who has been attending the Cardiology Clinic for several years and who has underlying atrial fibrillation, it is highly likely that these abnormalities are due to amiodarone toxicity. Amiodarone is a class III anti-arrhythmic, which is very effective in the management of supraventricular and ventricular tachycardia. It is, however, associated with several side-effects and complications:

- hyper- or hypothyroidism
- photosensitivity
- hepatitis
- peripheral neuropathy
- pulmonary fibrosis

- corneal microdeposits
- metallic taste in the mouth
- skin discoloration (slate-grey pigmentation)
- arrhythmias
- ataxia
- optic neuritis
- myopathy
- epididymitis
- nausea.

CCF is unlikely. Although right-sided heart failure may cause hepatitis and pulmonary oedema secondary to left-sided failure may cause a restrictive deficit and reduced transfer factor, CCF is unlikely in view of the echo. Also, this answer does not satisfactorily explain the patient's hyperthyroidism and skin discoloration. A chest infection would not account for the skin discoloration, blood tests or PFTs. Hyperthyroidism would not explain the patient's breathlessness, skin discoloration, hepatitis or PFTs. Hereditary haemochromatosis is an autosomal recessive disorder of iron metabolism, in which increased iron absorption leads to its deposition in multiple organs. It can cause bronze or slate-grey skin pigmentation, hepatitis, hepatomegaly and cirrhosis. In the heart it may cause a dilated cardiomyopathy and arrhythmias. It does not account for this patient's hyperthyroidism or PFTs.

1.23   E: Pituitary insufficiency

This woman has hypoglycaemia. Polycystic ovarian syndrome is associated with insulin resistance and therefore patients are more likely to develop diabetes mellitus (DM) or impaired glucose tolerance. In haemochromatosis, iron may accumulate in the pancreas, leading to insulin deficiency and secondary diabetes. Steroid therapy causes insulin resistance and thereby diabetes and impaired glucose tolerance. Metformin does not cause hypoglycaemia. Fasting hypoglycaemia may be caused by administration of insulin/sulphonylureas, insulinoma, alcohol (alcohol metabolism occurs at the expense of hepatic gluconeogenesis), Addison disease, pituitary insufficiency (due to impaired growth hormone and ACTH secretion), liver failure, non-pancreatic tumours (especially retroperitoneal sarcomas) or autoimmune hypoglycaemia (eg in Hodgkin disease). Insulin receptor antibodies normally cause insulin-resistant DM by blocking the insulin receptor. Rarely do they cause receptor activation with fasting hypoglycaemia. Anti-insulin antibodies cause accumulation of antibody-bound insulin, which then dissociates, resulting in high insulin levels. Post-prandial hypoglycaemia can occur post-gastrectomy.

1.24   E: Ethanol toxicity

This patient has a high anion gap acidosis. She also has a raised osmolal gap. The osmolal gap is the difference between the lab estimation of osmolality and the calculated osmolality. To calculate the plasma osmolality:

2([Na+]+[K+]) + [urea] + [glucose]

The osmolal gap is usually <10. If it is >10 consider: raised levels of alcohol, eg methanol, ethanol, ethylene glycol, isoprenolol, diethyleneglycol; diabetes mellitus; renal failure (retention of various organic and inorganic molecules). Type-2 RTA and Addison disease are associated with normal anion gap acidosis. Salicylate toxicity gives a high anion gap acidosis but does not produce a high osmolal gap. Conn syndrome causes a metabolic alkalosis.

1.25   B: Alkaptonuria (ochronosis)

This is a rare autosomal recessive disease. Homogentisic acid accumulates because of a deficiency in the enzyme homogentisic acid oxidase. The homogentisic acid polymerises to produce the black–brown alkapton, which is deposited in cartilage and connective tissue. Urine becomes dark on standing due to oxidation and polymerisation of homogentisic acid. Abnormal pigmentation is found in the ear and sclerae as well as articular cartilage. Premature arthritis occurs, predominantly affecting the spine and later the large joints. Intervertebral disc calcification is characteristic of alkaptonuria. The knees are commonly affected, although there is usually sparing of the sacro-iliac joints. The diagnosis is confirmed by checking a urinary homogentisic acid level. Homogentisic acid is a reducing substance and therefore gives a positive reaction to glucostix (Clinistix). Other causes of false-positive results are: fructose, pentose, lactose, salicylates, ascorbic acid.

1.26   C: Type-1 (distal) renal tube acidosis (RTA)

This patient has a hypokalaemic hyperchloraemic normal anion gap acidosis. Despite the severe systemic acidosis she has not acidified her urine. She has also had two vertebral crush fractures, an unusual occurrence without prior trauma in someone so young. In the context of the history it may suggest the presence of osteoporosis. The right loin pain suggests urinary tract infection or calculus. Type-1 RTA is typically severe (the bicarbonate may be reduced below 10 mmol/l). The basic defect is an inability to secrete protons in the distal tubule. This results in an inappropriate inability to acidify the urine below pH 5.3. Since H^+ reabsorption is abnormal, more sodium is reabsorbed, either with chloride or in exchange for potassium to maintain electroneutrality (hence the hyperchloraemia and hypokalaemia). Complications include osteoporosis, nephrocalcinosis and renal calculi. Growth failure and urinary tract infections may also occur. A renal calculus may be present, but this answer does not account for the history of fractures, the serum biochemistry and urinary pH. DKA does not cause a normal anion gap acidosis and would not lead to failure to acidify the urine. This answer also does not tie in with the history of vertebral fractures. A UTI may cause these symptoms and haematuria but does not explain the fractures, urinary pH or serum biochemistry. Type-2 (proximal) RTA typically causes a less severe acidosis (with a bicarbonate of 14–20 mmol/l). It causes osteomalacia and rickets rather than osteoporosis (due to phosphate wasting and reduced production of 1,25-dihydroxy vitamin D_3. The basic defect is proximal tubular bicarbonate wasting due to a resetting of the T_{max} of bicarbonate reabsorption. In the stable state bicarbonate wasting does not persist as the plasma bicarbonate stabilises at the concentration at which the proximal tubule is able to absorb all the filtered bicarbonate. Therefore the urine is typically appropriately acidified, especially in the morning. There may be other tubular abnormalities, such as glycosuria, aminoaciduria, uricosuria and phosphaturia.

1.27   B: Chronic liver disease occurs in 50–80% of those infected

Hepatitis C is an RNA virus. Interferon–γ results in clearance of the virus in only 25% of patients with chronic liver disease. It initially leads to normalisation of liver function and loss of HCV RNA in 50% of patients, although 6 months later 50% of these are positive again. Ribavirin is also used to treat chronic infection. Fulminant hepatitis is very rare. Transmission is by sexual contact or through contaminated blood.

1.28   D: Blood levels of HBeAg correlate with infectivity

HBeAg and HBV DNA correlate with viral replication and hence infectivity. The virus may be found in cell types other than hepatocytes, eg renal tubules, lymph nodes. This may partly explain recurrence after transplantation. Approximately 10% develop chronic infection. IgG HBcAb alone implies continuing viral replication. IgG HBcAb in low titres, together with HBsAb implies a previous, cleared infection. Patients who are immunodeficient are more likely to develop chronic viral hepatitis than those who are immunocompetent. Successful clearance of the virus is dependent on the cell-mediated immune response. The stronger the response, the more cells die and the higher the enzyme levels. The opposite occurs in immunocompromised patients. They are more likely to develop chronic disease.

1.29   E: Severe complications occur due to the production of an exotoxin that inhibits protein synthesis

This patient has diphtheria. This is caused by infection with *Corynebacterium diphtheriae,* an aerobic, non-invasive Gram-positive rod. The organism produces an exotoxin that inhibits protein synthesis and causes local tissue destruction and membrane formation. It affects all cells but its most prominent effects are seen in the heart (where it causes myocarditis), nerves (where it leads to demyelination) and kidneys (where it produces tubular necrosis). Disease may involve almost any mucous membrane.The most common sites of infection are the pharynx and tonsils. Patients usually present with malaise, a sore throat, anorexia and a low-grade fever. Within 2 to 3 days a membrane forms and extends. The larynx may be involved, leading to hoarseness, a barking cough and, in some cases, airway obstruction. Severe complications are due to the toxin. The severity of these is usually proportional to the severity of the local disease. Myocarditis may lead to heart failure and arrhythmias. Neurological complications mainly affect motor nerves. Local paralysis with paralysis of the soft palate and involvement of other cranial nerves may occur in the first few days. A peripheral neuritis, principally motor, may occur later. This usually begins proximally and extends distally. Respiratory failure and pneumonia may result. Treatment should be begun as soon as a presumptive diagnosis is made. This consists of diphtheria antitoxin, erythromycin, isolation and supportive management. Close contacts should receive prophylactic antibiotics and a diphtheria booster.

1.30   D: An overdose of diazepam

The patient in the question has type-II respiratory failure: hypoxia ($p_a(O_2) < 8$ kPa) with a raised $p_a(CO_2)$ (>6.5 kPa). Type-II respiratory failure results from alveolar hypoventilation with or without ventilation/perfusion (V/Q) mismatch. Causes include:

- thoracic wall disease, eg kyphoscoliosis, flail chest, ankylosing spondylitis
- neurological disorders, eg Guillain–Barré, multiple sclerosis, polio, motor neurone disease, cervical cord lesion
- muscular disease, eg myasthenia gravis, muscular dystrophy
- sedative drugs
- pulmonary disease, eg COPD, late stages of severe asthma, emphysema, pulmonary fibrosis.

Type-I respiratory failure is defined as hypoxia ($p_a(O_2) < 8$ kPa) with a low or normal $p_a(CO_2)$. It is caused primarily by V/Q mismatch. Causes of type-I respiratory failure include: pulmonary embolism, pneumonia, asthma, pulmonary oedema, pulmonary haemorrhage, pneumothorax, adult respiratory distress syndrome, fibrosing alveolitis, emphysema.

1.31 B: Approximately 95% of the subjects have systolic blood pressures between 101 and 189 mmHg

The distribution of systolic blood pressure is normal or Gaussian, because the mean and median values are equal. Therefore, 95% of observations fall within two standard deviations (not standard errors) of the mean or between 101 and 189 mmHg; 2.5% of the subjects will have a systolic blood pressure greater than 189 mmHg. Approximately 68% of the values lie within one standard deviation of the mean, ie between 123 and 167 mmHg and 99% of the observations fall within 2.6 standard deviations (SD) of the mean.

1.32 C: The statistical significance of the fall in blood glucose may be analysed by a paired Student's *t*-test

A paired *t*-test could be used to compare the means of the blood glucose in patients before and after administration of the new drug. This is a parametrical test, which assumes that the data are normally distributed. Non-parametrical tests should be used when the data has a skewed distribution or when data is qualitative. Examples of non-parametrical tests include the Mann–Whitney *U*-test, chi-squared test, Kendall's S score and the Wilcoxon rank sum test. Conventionally, a value of $P < 0.05$ is taken to be statistically significant, ie there is less than a 1 in 20 chance that there is no significant difference between the two groups, so allowing the null hypothesis to be rejected. If the *P* value = 0.01, 1 in 100 studies would be expected to show a significant effect of the drug on blood glucose by chance alone. If $P = 0.05$, there is a 1 in 20 chance that a significant difference in blood glucose would occur by chance alone. In a double-blind study neither the researcher nor the patient knows which treatment the patient has been randomised to receive. In a single-blind study either the patient or the doctor does not know (usually the patient).

1.33 B: Cortisol binds to the mineralocorticoid receptor

Thyroid hormone binds to two receptors, the α and β thyroid hormone receptors. These are members of the nuclear receptor family and are intracellular. Cortisol binds to both the glucocorticoid and mineralocorticoid receptors with high affinity. ACTH receptors are expressed on the adrenal gland and are G protein coupled. PPAR-γ is essential for adipocyte differentiation and is the target of the thioridazine group of glitazone drugs. Insulin causes dimerisation of its receptors and then activates tyrosine kinase activity within the receptor.

1.34 B: Graves disease is associated with myasthenia gravis

Toxic multi-nodular goitre is unlikely to respond to antithyroid drugs in the long term and is an indication for surgery or radioiodine. Graves disease is associated with other autoimmune diseases, including myasthenia gravis. Carbimazole is not contraindicated in pregnancy, but propylthiouracil is usually used as there are anecdotal accounts of aplasia cutis in the offspring of carbimazole-treated mothers. Smoking is a risk factor for development of Graves ophthalmopathy and also predicts worsening of the eye disease after radioactive iodine. Radioactive iodine may exacerbate ophthalmic Graves disease.

1.35 A: Amiodarone

Renal failure causes hypogonadism and so gynaecomastia. Klinefelter syndrome (47,XXY) also causes hypogonadism. Spironolactone increases sex hormone-binding globulin and so reduces available androgen. As a result, oestrogen acts unopposed on the breast and causes gynaecomastia. Amiodarone affects the thyroid gland and is not associated with gynaecomastia. Testicular or adrenal cancers can produce oestrogen and so cause gynaecomastia.

1.36 A: 90% of patients respond to long-acting somatostatin analogue treatment

Around 90% of patients will respond to long-acting somatostatin therapy. Microadenomas have a 90% cure rate in experienced surgical centres. Macroadenomas (>10 mm in diameter) have a lower cure rate of < 40%. Suprasellar extension does not preclude a trans-sphenoidal approach. The local anatomy of the tumour is important and is the indication (eg decompression of the optic chiasm). Diabetes occurs in >10% of acromegalic patients. Hypercholesterolaemia is not associated with acromegaly, but cardiovascular disease and increased mortality are.

1.37 B: They are made using human B lymphocytes

Monoclonal antibodies are made by fusing a mouse B cell expressing a specific antibody with a mouse myeloma cell line. The myeloma cells give the B cells immortality and the resulting hybridoma can be grown in vitro indefinitely. The antibodies produced can be purified and used in radioimmunoassays to measure hormones, can be used in histology to look for expression of specific proteins and can be used therapeutically and in vitro to activate T lymphocytes.

1.38   C: They cause 'ragged red' fibres in skeletal muscle

The mitochondrial genome is small and circular. It is exclusively inherited from the mother (sperm contain no mitochondria). The genome is vulnerable to mutations and inheritance of some mutated mitochondrial chromosomes increases the likelihood of developing disease. The tissues characteristically involved are muscle, brain, nerve and pancreatic islet. Encephalopathy, myopathy, diabetes and lactic acidosis are characteristic features.

1.39   E: It results from amplification of triplet repeats within genes

Genetic anticipation results from the amplification of unstable triplet base repeats within the coding region of genes within affected families. As a result, the size of the repeat increases with successive generations and so the age of onset of disease declines. Huntington disease and fragile-X syndrome are both examples. Turner syndrome cannot be inherited and is a chromosomal loss disease.

1.40   D: RNA polymerase II gives rise to protein encoding mRNA

Mammalian mRNA is monocistronic (ie each mRNA encodes one protein), in contrast to bacterial mRNA. RNA polymerase II is responsible for transcribing mRNA. Introns are transcribed and then spliced out of the RNA to give mature mRNA before the mRNA leaves the nucleus. The genetic code is degenerate and so multiple codons (triplets of nucleotides) encode the same amino acid. Therefore, not all changes in the nucleotide sequence will give rise to changes in the protein sequence. Usually about 1% of cellular RNA is mRNA; the rest is structural.

1.41   A: Activates the NFκB transcription factor

Tumour necrosis factor-α (TNF-α) can bind a p55 and a p75 receptor. The receptors are coupled to death pathways and so can induce apoptosis in susceptible cells. TNF-α induces activation of NFκB. TNF-α has been linked with insulin resistance, especially in obesity. TNF-α is elevated in synovial fluid and anti-TNF is useful in treating rheumatoid arthritis. TNF-α induces expression of other proinflammatory cytokines, including IL-1 and IL-6.

1.42   D: Progression from predominantly small peripheral joint disease to involve more proximal, larger joints

Rheumatoid arthritis is a multi-factorial disease with an important genetic component. Approximately 20% of identical twins will develop the disease.

HLA class II antigen DR4 is associated with disease and the association is stronger with more severe disease (ie seropositivity; > 70% of seropositive patients are DR4 positive). The typical progression is from peripheral small joints to later involvement of the larger joints, but sacroiliac disease is rare.

1.43   D: Patients have a characteristic reduction in circulating CD8$^+$ T lymphocytes

Polymyalgia rheumatica (PMR) is a disorder of middle aged and elderly patients. Disease is rare before age 45 or after age 80. A third of patients are aged < 60 years. The onset is rapid, with full development in a month. Systemic features include weight loss, night sweats, fever, fatigue and malaise and are common. Muscle enzymes and EMG are normal in PMR. Patients respond rapidly to prednisolone, but so do patients with sepsis, osteoarthritis and rheumatoid arthritis and so the improvement is not helpful for diagnosis. There is a characteristic loss of CD8$^+$ T cytotoxic/suppressor cells which can persist up to a year after clinical remission.

1.44   E: Over-represented in Whipple disease

HLA-B27 is a class I HLA or major histocompatibility complex (MHC) antigen and is expressed on most cells types. It is over-represented in ankylosing spondylitis (90% of patients compared to 8% of normals), Whipple disease, reactive arthritis, psoriatic arthritis, Reiter syndrome and uveitis. It is not over-represented in Crohn disease, ulcerative colitis or Behçet disease. Class II HLA antigens are expressed on antigen-presenting cells, like dendritic cells and B lymphocytes.

1.45   D: High frequencies of disease are seen in women of Chinese ancestry

Systemic lupus erythematosus (SLE) is commoner in women with African, Chinese, Asian or South American Indian ancestry, compared to North Europeans. Women are affected more frequently than men (9:1) and there is an increased incidence in Klinefelter syndrome (47,XXY). The skin is a target organ in 70% of cases. Around 15% of the normal population have Raynaud's phenomenon; in SLE the incidence is between 20% and 30%. C-reactive protein is not raised in SLE.

1.46   C: Hyaline casts consist of Tamm–Horsfall protein

Hyaline casts are made of Tamm–Horsfall protein, a mucoprotein secreted by the distal convoluted tubule. They are found in normal urine, more so after exercise, during febrile illness and after loop diuretics. Oxalate crystals are found in normal urine if it is allowed to stand. When present in freshly passed urine or in large amounts, they indicate a predisposition to stone formation. Cystine crystals indicate cystinuria. Counts of >10 white cells per ml urine is abnormal, usually indicating urinary tract infection. A few red cells are found in normal urine; >2000 cells per ml is probably abnormal.

1.47   A: Aciclovir

The clearance of a drug depends on size and protein binding. Most antibiotics are small and so are dialysed, with the exception of vancomycin, amphotericin and erythromycin. Protein-bound drugs like warfarin and propranolol are not cleared.

1.48   D: Urine sodium > 20 mmol/l

Pre-renal failure is caused by poor renal perfusion. The kidney retains sodium (hence urine sodium concentrations are low) and excretes urea (hence urine urea concentrations are high compared to plasma). The urine osmolality is high. Associated features of hypovolaemia should be sought and these include postural hypotension and decreased pulmonary wedge pressures.

1.49   B: Abdominal pain is a common presenting feature

The inheritance is autosomal dominant. Abdominal pain, spontaneous haematuria, an increase in girth, hypertension, urinary tract infection, renal colic and renal impairment may all be presenting features of this disease. There is no specific treatment for the condition, which will require renal replacement therapy between ages 30 and 50 in most cases. A third of patients will have a hepatic cyst and a few pancreatic or splenic cysts. Berry aneurysms in the cerebral circulation may cause haemorrhage in approximately 10% of patients.

1.50   E: The proximal nephron actively secretes hydrogen ions, in contrast to the distal nephron

Under normal circumstances both the proximal and distal tubule actively secrete hydrogen ions into the tubular fluid. These combine with filtered bicarbonate ions to form carbonic acid, which dissociates into water and carbon dioxide. The carbon dioxide is reabsorbed and used to generate bicarbonate ions, which are returned to the circulation. Approximately 90% of the bicarbonate ions filtered by the glomerulus are recovered in this manner. In distal renal tubular acidosis there is a mild chronic hyperchloraemic metabolic acidosis (normal anion gap), with exacerbations of acidosis. There is failure of the distal tubule to secrete hydrogen ions and so the urine pH seldom falls below 5.5. About 70% of patients will have nephrocalcinosis or renal calculi, distinguishing the disorder from the other renal tubular acidoses. Proximal tubular acidosis is rare as an isolated defect and is often found with amino-aciduria, glycosuria, hyperphosphaturia and uricosuria. The condition is usually part of a Fanconi syndrome but may result from poisoning (eg outdated tetracycline).

1.51   D: It is a lentivirus

HIV is a lentivirus (a virus with slow progression). There are two forms, 1 and 2. Both forms cause AIDS, but disease progression is slower with type-2. The two viruses appear to have distinct evolutionary origins. The HIV viruses are retroviruses, with RNA-containing genomes. HIV gains entry to the cell via a chemokine receptor and results in depletion of CD4 cells. An adverse indicator is elevation of the CD8 cell count.

1.52   B: Pneumococcal otitis media is usually associated with neutrophil leucocytosis

Pneumococcus is a Gram-positive organism. Pneumococcal pneumonia shows a peak in winter, probably due to low humidity, low temperature and respiratory virus infection. Otitis media due to *Pneumococcus* is usually associated with neutrophilia, which can be helpful in diagnosis. Pneumococcal meningitis is accompanied by a high mortality rate, even with modern treatment. The disease carries a mortality at least five times greater than that of meningococcal meningitis. Sickle cell disease results in hyposplenism and so predisposes to pneumococcal disease, which can be prevented by antibody prophylaxis.

1.53   D: Herpes meningitis is a relatively benign condition in adults

Herpes simplex consists of two types: 1, which mainly causes orofacial disease; and 2, which mainly causes genital disease. Herpes meningitis is benign, with normal adults recovering in about a week; no specific treatment is needed. Erythaema multiforme frequently results from previous herpes infection. Antibody titres are only useful in retrospective diagnosis on the basis of a rising titre in the convalescent phase. The herpes viruses are double-stranded DNA viruses.

1.54 B: Identification of Gram-positive diplococci on lumbar puncture suggests meningococcal meningitis

Meningococci are Gram-negative diplococci. Acute septicaemia is associated with neutrophilia, as is meningitis; leucopenia is rarely found in fulminating cases. The classic early skin lesion is a petechial rash, but as the condition deteriorates more extensive haemorrhagic lesions develop. Rifampicin eradicates nasal carriage of meningococci in 25% at 6 days and 19% at 2 weeks. Transmission is usually by respiratory droplet, though sexual transmission is also reported.

1.55 A: Aortic dissection is a recognised complication

Mutations in Marfan syndrome are scattered throughout the gene on chromosome 15 that encodes fibrillin, a component of microfibrils in the extracellular matrix. The mutations are most often missense, that is, they result in an amino acid substitution. The gene contains 65 exons. Marfan syndrome is inherited in an autosomal dominant fashion with variable expression but generally full penetrance. New mutations occur in about 15–30% of cases. Slit lamp examination is required for detection of slight lens dislocation.

ANSWERS

Infectious Diseases

INFECTIOUS DISEASES 'BEST OF FIVE' ANSWERS

2.1   B: Histoplasmosis

Marked elevation of LDH, coupled with the diagnosis of HIV/AIDs and the respiratory features seen here is highly suggestive of infiltration with histoplasmosis. The anaemia and raised LFTs also fit with this picture. Histoplasmosis is prevalent in the USA and tropical regions of Africa and Asia. Diagnosis is usually made via urinary antigen testing and the treatment is iv amphotericin B.

2.2   D: Primigravida women appear the most at risk from infection

Primigravida women appear the most at risk from infection. Pregnant women are said to be 10 times more likely to suffer from malaria, with infection being more severe as well. Out of these women, primigravida are said to be the most at risk of all. Quinine and quinidine are not recommended in pregnancy, although the benefits for chloroquine and primaquine probably outweigh the risks of use.

2.3   B: It increases pH in intracellular organelles and may interact with parasite DNA

It increases pH in intracellular organelles and may interact with parasite DNA. Chloroquine, primaquine and quinine all are thought to lead to increasing pH within parasitic acid vesicles. In addition, they have variable levels of interaction and binding to parasitic DNA. Tetracycline-based antibiotics and clindamycin block parasitic ribosomal activity.

2.4   C: Human papillomavirus (HPV) subtypes 6 and 11 commonly cause this infection

HPV subtypes 6 and 11 are a common cause of genital warts. HPV subtypes 16 and 18 are most strongly associated with the development of cervical cancer, so as such infection with 6 and 11 does not greatly increase the risk of the disease. A vaccine has been developed with activity against 6, 11, 16 and 18 and has now become a part of the vaccination schedule for girls in a number of countries. Spontaneous regression of warts is common, as is recurrence and biopsy is not a usual part of the diagnostic schedule.

2.5   B: Epidemics in young people were often due to the 'C' type

Epidemics in the late teenage population were historically due to *Neisseria meningitides* type C, however after a vaccination programme the number of cases is rapidly diminishing. Unfortunately, no vaccine against type B exists, although a number of candidates are in development. Some resistance to penicillin exists, so that cerebrospinal fluid (CSF) penetrating cephalosporins are now seen as the treatment of choice. Rifampicin is standard prophylaxis for contacts of patients infected with meningococcus.

2.6   A: Penicillin im is the treatment of choice

This patient has the classic presentation of primary syphilis; penicillin is usually given as a single dose of 2.4 million units im, as the tendency of patients not to return to the clinic and lack of patient compliance means that multiple dose courses of medication are often not followed. Unfortunately, new cases of syphilis infection are increasing in younger patients. This man should supply the names of sexual contacts and consider an HIV test.

2.7   A: *Candida albicans*

The big clues as to the diagnosis are the history of type 1 diabetes and the fact that his diabetes is currently poorly controlled. While his history of unprotected sex may prompt screening for sexually transmitted diseases, a sexually transmitted cause of his symptoms is unlikely here. Improved glycaemic control is an essential part of his management, treatment for the *Candida* infection includes topical co-trimoxazole or a single dose of fluconazole.

2.8   B: Bacterial vaginosis

The amine-like smell to the vaginal discharge, increased vaginal pH and presence of clue cells are clear hints as to the diagnosis. No active treatment is required for the condition; the best advice is to avoid washing the vulval area with soaps and cleansing with water. Lactic acid containing vulval washes may be of use in reducing the chance of future infection.

2.9   D: Another member of the class has been terminated due to hepatotoxicity

Aplaviroc, under development by GSK was terminated due to hepatotoxicity. Maraviroc is a CCR5 inhibitor, CCR5 is a natural chemokine receptor that HIV uses to allow entry to macrophages. Natural ligands of the CCR5 receptor include RANTES, MIP-1α and MIP-1β. CCR5 is expressed predominantly on T cells, macrophages, dendritic cells and microglia. It is thought that use of CCR5 inhibitors might cause HIV mutations to evolve which gain entry to cells via a co-receptor, but this has not become apparent.

2.10   E: The virus was first identified in Hong Kong

H5N1 was first identified in Hong Kong in 1997. Currently human-to-human transmission is thought to be very unlikely and those who work in close proximity to poultry are most at risk of infection. Currently a higher level of resistance to oseltamivir versus zanamivir has been identified. Oseltamivir is also thought to be associated with an increased risk of psychiatric side-effects. Candidate vaccines against H5N1 are currently under development.

2.11   B: *Chlamydia trachomatis*

This patient gives symptoms consistent with pelvic inflammatory disease and from the options given, *Chlamydia* infection is the most likely diagnosis. Cell culture for *Chlamydia* is difficult; therefore, serology forms the mainstay of diagnosis. Typical antibiotics used for treating *Chlamydia* infection include doxycycline and azithromycine, as a one-week or single course respectively. Unfortunately, one case series suggested up to 40% of patients with PID may be misdiagnosed, risking the possibility of long-term fertility problems.

2.12   B: Genotype 1 accounts for between 40 and 80% of hepatitis C cases

Genotype 1 is the commonest genotype associated with hepatitis C cases, it responds to antiviral therapy less well than types 2 and 3 and therefore requires treatment for at least 1 year. Liver biopsy in hepatitis C infection usually demonstrates lymphocytic infiltration and in advanced cases features consistent with cirrhosis. Pegylated interferon therapy combined with ribavirin is the mainstay of treatment. Hepatocellular carcinoma develops an average of 30 years after infection.

2.13   C: The risk of transmission to the child is around 90%

In patients who are HBeAg positive, transmission rates are around 90%. Where eAg is negative, transmission rates are only around 10–40%. Around 95% of transmissions occur intrapartum. Chronic hepatitis B is associated with less than 0.2% of pregnancies. Where acute infection occurs it tends to be less severe when associated with pregnancy. Active or passive immunisation is very effective at reducing transmission rates.

2.14   A: Prion protein is encoded on the host genome

Prion protein is encoded on the host genome and the amino acid sequence varies between species. Normal prion protein is produced and cleared in normal individuals. Abnormal prion protein, however, accumulates, leading to plaque formation surrounded by spongiform change. Glycosylation patterns are similar between BSE prion protein and vCJD prion protein. Patients homozygous for methionine or valine at codon 129 of the prion protein are at greater risk of more rapid disease progression. Infectivity of abnormal prion protein can be reduced and abolished by proteolytic enzymes, but not by standard sterilisation or nucleases. Tonsillar biopsy is useful in the diagnosis of variant CJD but not sporadic CJD.

2.15   D: Yellow fever vaccine

Yellow fever vaccine is a live attenuated vaccine and has caused fatal disease in patients with very advanced HIV disease. Small studies have suggested that it is probably sage in patients whose HIV is not advanced. The other vaccines are either killed or subunit vaccines. Their efficacy is very much lower in patients with advanced HIV but they are otherwise safe.

2.16   E: Hepatitis C

The list of statutory notifiable diseases can be found in the British National Formulary. There are many surprising omissions from this list, which appears rather out of date. Viral hepatitis is the only one of the five answers given that is on the list.

2.17   D: Rectal biopsy

This man has schistosomiasis, which is endemic in the great lakes of Africa. Some six weeks after exposure patients may develop a fever, eosinophilia and urticaria (Katayama fever). At this time patients infected with *Schistosoma mansoni* may develop a frank colitis due to a vigorous granulomatous reaction around the eggs making their way out through the wall of the colon. Diagnosis is by microscopy for ova, either in the stool for *S. mansoni* or urine for *S. haematobium*. Eggs of either species may be seen by low-power microscopy of rectal biopsies. Antibodies against *Schistosoma* species can be detected but may take up to three months from exposure to develop. The drug of choice is praziquantel.

African trypanosomiasis (*Trypanosoma brucei* var. *rhodesiense* or *gambiense*) is transmitted by the bite of the tsetse fly and causes an acute febrile illness and subsequently sleeping sickness. There is no eosinophilia. Amoebic dysentery and amoebic liver abscesses cause a neutrophilia. Filarial infections do cause an eosinophilia, but not bloody diarrhoea.

2.18 B: Doxycycline

He has African tick typhus (*Rickettsia africae*) which is an extremely common infection, particularly among visitors to game parks. Sero-epidemiological studies of local people show extremely high rates of past infection. Typically, a black scab (eschar) forms at the site of the tick bite, the patient becomes febrile and complains of a severe headache and may develop a very sparse maculo-papular rash. The condition is normally self-limiting but the clinical course is shortened by treatment with doxycycline. Diagnosis is usually made by testing acute and convalescent sera for a rise in specific antibody titre. Culture of the organism is hazardous for laboratory staff. Praziquantel is used in the treatment of schistosomiasis, sodium stibogluconate for leishmaniasis and melarsoprol for African trypanosomiasis.

2.19 B: *Chlamydia trachomatis*

This man has urethritis, presumably of infectious origin. Recurrent herpes simplex can occasionally affect the urethra. The negative Gram stain does not exclude gonorrhoea but it is more likely that he has non-specific urethritis (non-gonococcal urethritis), the commonest cause of which is *C. trachomatis*. It is unlikely that a primary syphilitic chancre would cause urethritis and it is likely it would be noticed on examination. Although he claims to be mono-gamous, his partner may not be.

2.20 D: Yellow fever

All of these illnesses are transmitted by the bite of a mosquito. Yellow fever is present in South America and sub-Saharan Africa, but is not present in Asia or Southeast Asia although the mosquito vectors of these areas seem capable of transmitting it in experimental situations. Dengue fever causes huge epidemics in the tropics and is frequently seen as a cause of fever in the returning traveller. *W. bancrofti* and *P. vivax* are widely distributed throughout the tropics. Japanese encephalitis has a wide distribution throughout Asia.

2.21 E: Persistent, uncontrolled infection can occur as an X-linked condition in males

This is acute Epstein–Barr virus (EBV) infection. Persistent uncontrolled EBV infection does occur very rarely and can be diagnosed by detecting high levels of EBV DNA in the blood. It is presumed that these patients have a hitherto unsuspected immunological deficit leading to the failure to control the virus. X-linked proliferative syndrome (XLP, Duncan syndrome) is a congenital syndrome of failure to control EBV. The atypical lymphocytes are CD8 T lymphocytes. The Paul–Bunnell test detects the presence of heterophile antibodies that do not appear to be directed against any EBV antigens. The tonsillar enlargement may be severe enough to cause respiratory embarrassment and should be treated with intravenous steroids. A fine maculopapular rash is very common. A much more dramatic rash is seen when the patient is given amoxicillin (including in co-amoxiclav) or ampicillin, which should therefore be avoided.

2.22   D: The illness is highly unlikely to be acute pulmonary histoplasmosis

Although this woman is from the right area of the USA to have contracted histoplasmosis, the incubation period of acute pulmonary histoplasmosis is one to three weeks. Blood cultures are only positive in 10–30% of patients with *S. pneumoniae* pneumonia, pneumococcal urinary antigen detection being a much more sensitive test. Serology for any acute respiratory infection is likely to be negative early in illness and is best detected some two to four weeks after the onset of symptoms. *Legionella* urinary antigen testing only detects *Legionella pneumophila* type 1, which does account for 70% or more of infections. Cold agglutinins (detectable at the bedside by cooling blood in an EDTA bottle and then examining visually for red cell agglutination) are virtually diagnostic of *Mycoplasma*, the only other common condition producing cold agglutinins at this level being non-Hodgkin lymphoma.

2.23   A: Brucellosis

Brucellosis is caused by a Gram-negative coccobacillus, which grows reasonably quickly by modern blood culture techniques. *Coxiella burnetii* (the causative agent of Q fever) does not grow in blood culture. RVF and CCHF are both viral infections transmitted by direct blood contact and possibly also by mosquitoes (RVF) and tick bites (CCHF). In acute sleeping sickness (*Trypanosoma brucei* var. *gambiense* or *rhodesiense*) the trypanosomes are often visible on a thick blood film, but sleeping sickness does not occur in the Middle East. The other four illnesses do occur, especially in people in close contact with herds of sheep and goats, with brucellosis and Q fever being more common than the other two diseases.

2.24   A: *Candida albicans*

Prolonged stay in an intensive care unit is associated with an increased risk of *Candida* septicaemia and this is by far the most likely diagnosis. Cryptococci are also sometimes grown from blood culture. *Histoplasma* and *Coccidioides* may also be grown from blood culture in disseminated disease, but are not present in the UK.

2.25   D: Continue all medication and repeat liver function tests in one week

A degree of hepatitis is almost invariable with tuberculosis (TB) medication but it is rarely a clinical problem. Rifampicin, isoniazid and pyrazinamide are all hepatotoxic. (Ethambutol causes optic neuritis.) The British Thoracic Society recommendations for the treatment of tuberculosis suggest continuing therapy and weekly monitoring of patients if the transaminases are between two and five times the upper limit of normal. TB medication should be discontinued if the transaminases are above five times the upper limit of normal and gradually re-introduced when the liver function tests have improved. It is important not to undertreat TB or to use a single agent as that increases the likelihood of treatment failure and the development of drug resistance.

2.26   D: Enhanced antimycobacterial immune reaction

This woman has developed an immune reconstitution inflammatory syndrome (IRIS). It is commonly seen and is probably due to recovery of the immune system (due to the antiretrovirals) to a level where the immune system is able to recognise antigens of infectious agents that it had previously failed to recognise. It usually presents with painful enlargement of lymph nodes in the case of TB or *Mycobacterium avium intracellulare* infection and is associated with fever and an increase in inflammatory markers. (IRIS can occur to antigens of other organisms, eg CMV.) Once the clinician is confident that there is no other infection, it is usually treated with a low-dose of steroids.

2.27   A: Request sequencing of his HIV to look for mutations indicating resistance to antiretroviral drugs

It is likely that this man's HIV has developed resistance mutations to his current antiretroviral regime. Detection of resistance mutations by sequencing is now routine practice and is strongly recommended to guide any change of medication in a patient failing therapy, rather than attempting a best guess. Adding a single new agent is bound to fail as resistance will develop extremely rapidly. Poor compliance with therapy is more likely to lead to the development of resistant virus. It is always worth rechecking the CD4 count and HIV viral load as these assays are sometimes subject to laboratory error. His CD4 count is less than 200 × 10⁶/l. He is therefore at risk of developing *Pneumocystis carinii* pneumonia and should be started on prophylactic co-trimoxazole, but prophylaxis against MAI is not routinely given if the CD4 count is greater than 100 × 10⁶/l. The measurement of p24 antigen has no place in routine monitoring – it is merely a less sensitive way than RT-PCR of detecting the presence of virus.

2.28   B: Bone marrow aspirate

The differential diagnosis is quite wide and includes tuberculosis, lymphoma, HIV and visceral leishmaniasis (kala-azar). (Southern Sudan has been experiencing a continuing epidemic of visceral leishmaniasis for over 15 years.) A bone marrow aspirate will allow culture for tuberculosis (TB) and leishmaniasis and microscopy for lymphoma, TB and leishmaniasis and will probably give more information than any of the other tests. A liver biopsy (transjugular in view of the thrombocytopenia) would also probably help, but would be less good for the diagnosis of leishmaniasis. Mantoux testing is insensitive in very ill patients (high false-negative rate) and rarely helpful in this situation. Slit skin smears are used for diagnosing cutaneous leishmaniasis and leprosy.

2.29   A: Parvovirus B19

Parvovirus B19 causes a chronic anaemia in immunocompromised patients by causing a persistent infection affecting the erythroblasts. It is spread by the respiratory route and is associated with respiratory symptoms but has only rarely been reported to be associated with any major respiratory problems. It responds to intravenous immunoglobulin, which may have to be given repeatedly in patients who fail to eradicate it due to their immunocompromised state.

2.30   B: Quinine

The patient should receive intravenous quinine as soon as possible. Atovaquone/proguanil combination therapy is appropriate for uncomplicated, nonsevere *Plasmodium falciparum*. (Artemether and artesunate are at least as effective as quinine in the treatment of *falciparum* malaria and are in use in areas of quinine resistance in combination with other antimalarial drugs.) Exchange transfusion is suggested for patients with a parasitaemia of more than 30% (or more than 10% with complications) but it has never been subjected to a randomised controlled trial and evidence of efficacy has been obtained from retrospective studies and case reports. Haemofiltration, along with other supportive care is appropriate for established renal failure. *Plasmodium falciparum* malaria resistance to chloroquine is now world-wide and chloroquine should therefore never be used as a treatment option in the UK.

2.31   B:Leptospirosis

The combination of renal failure, jaundice without liver failure and a haemorrhagic conjunctivitis is highly suggestive of leptospirosis (acquired through direct water contact). Deaths tend to occur from myocarditis, overwhelming pulmonary haemorrhage and the complications of renal failure. Scrub typhus causes a debilitating fever and rash, sometimes with central nervous system (CNS) involvement. Melioidosis is an extremely common, typical Gram-negative septicaemic illness in the Far East and is acquired through water contact. (It can also cause a more prolonged, less severe illness.) Malaria must always be excluded in any traveller returning from an endemic area, but much of Thailand, including the main tourist areas but excepting the Thai borders, is free of malaria.

2.32   A: Acute HBV infection

Hepatitis B surface antigen (HBsAg) is an early indicator of acute infection. If it persists for more than six months in the presence of IgG antibodies to the core (anti-HBc IgG) it would suggest a chronic carrier state. Antibodies to HBsAg indicate recovery and immunity and are found after successful immunisation.

Anti-HBc IgM appear early in infection and persist during acute infection. The IgG subclass persists for life and indicates previous exposure to the hepatitis B virus. The 'e' antigen is associated with infectivity and is usually present for three to six weeks, rising and falling within the time span of a raised HBsAg. A persistent 'e' antigen would suggest a chronic carrier status.

2.33   E: Rotavirus

The options are all examples of human RNA viruses. Rotavirus infection occurs mainly in childhood and is associated with respiratory symptoms and diarrhoea. Arboviruses include yellow fever and dengue; arena viruses, Lassa fever and epidemic haemorrhagic fever. Picornavirus is associated with haemorrhagic conjunctivitis. An atypical form of measles, a paramyxovirus, is associated with severe illness and haemorrhage.

2.34   D: Melarsoprol is effective treatment

African trypanosomiasis follows the bite of the tsetse fly and the transfer of *T. brucei*. Humans are an important reservoir for the protozoan. The Rhodesian and Gambian forms of the disease are similar clinically except that Rhodesian sleeping sickness tends to be acute and severe rather than chronic and indolent and death from Rhodesian disease often occurs within one year. Fever, lymphadenopathy, hepatosplenomegaly and central nervous system (CNS) disease are common features. Suramin and pentamidine are useful therapies but do not cross the blood–brain barrier. CNS disease is best treated with melarsoprol but it is not effective in Rhodesian sleeping sickness.

2.35　B: *Plasmodium falciparum*

In humans, the malaria life cycle starts with the injection of the infective sporozoite through the skin by the Anopheles mosquito. During pre-erythrocytic schizogony sporozoites mature to micromerozoites in the liver and are then liberated into the bloodstream and infect red blood cells. It is in the ensuing erythrocytic stage that micromerozoites transform through a trophozoite and schizont phase to become the 'asexual' merozoites that are typically seen on a blood film. Some of these merozoites develop into 'sexual' gametocytes and at this stage the patient becomes infective.

A fourth exoerythrocytic phase exists. This occurs in the liver. A variable number of original sporozoites remain latent in the liver, not transforming to micromerozoites. In this way there appears to be a cycle of continuous re-infection. This phenomenon is definitely seen with *P. vivax*, probably occurs with *P. ovale* and possibly occurs with *P. malariae*. It is not a feature of the life cycle of P. *falciparum*. It is for this reason that primaquine is required for the eradication of *P. vivax*, *P. ovale* and *P. malariae*, as it has an effect on the exoerythrocytic cycle.

2.36　A: Cysticercosis

Cysticercosis occurs after ingesting the eggs of *Taenia solium* (pork tapeworm). It is seen in areas of Asia, Africa and South America. Cysterci may develop in any tissue of the body but are most commonly found as space-occupying cerebral lesions and subcutaneous nodules. Retinitis, uveitis, conjunctivitis, choroidal atrophy and blindness may also occur. The treatment of choice is praziquantel.

2.37　B: All of the options

Any impairment of host immunity, including chronic alcohol abuse, may add to the risk of an atypical infection. Healthy adults are usually immune, having developed capsular and specific bacteria-related antibodies, either directly related to *Haemophilus* exposure or through cross-reactivity with other common Gram-negative bacteria.

2.38   D: Leptospirosis

Infectious mononucleosis should be considered but the clinical features and risk associated with occupation point towards the spirochaetal infection, leptospirosis (Weil disease). The early, leptospiraemic phase is characterised by constitutional symptoms of fever, malaise, weight loss and headache. Infrequently there may be a rash, lymphadenopathy, or hepatosplenomegaly. During the second phase of the infection, 50% of patients complain of meningism. Most cases will resolve spontaneously but a small number develop renal impairment, haematuria, haemolytic anaemia, jaundice and cardiac failure.

The organism can be cultured from blood or cerebrospinal fluid in the first week. Serological tests for IgM antibodies are useful. Penicillin or erythromycin is a suitable treatment.

2.39   D: None of the options

Epidermolytic toxins of *S. aureus* cause scalded skin syndrome. This is indistinguishable from toxic epidermal necrolysis, which has a number of additional causes. However, given the number of staphylococcal infections, the association is uncommon. Toxic shock syndrome is mediated by toxins TSST1 and enterotoxins B and C; bacteraemia is rare and treatment is mainly supportive, though antibiotics are required to eradicate the focal source. A rapid onset of septicaemia is an infrequent complication of streptococcal cellulitis. Group A β-haemolytic *Streptococcus pyogenes* is associated with erysipelas in the elderly. Impetigo is usually superficial, not affecting the dermis. Ecthyma is an ulcerating form of impetigo, extending into the dermis. Both forms are associated with increased risk of glomerulonephritis.

2.40   A: All of the options

Atypical infections might also include *Nocardia, Candida, Mycoplasma, Mycobacterium*, cytomegalovirus, *Aspergillus* and *Pneumocystis*.

2.41   D: *Staphylococcus aureus* endocarditis and septicaemia

This is a description of *Staphylococcus aureus* septicaemia, tricuspid endocarditis and septic pulmonary emboli in an intravenous drug user. Confusion is common in severe sepsis and does not always indicate intracranial infection, although this must always be considered. *Streptococcus bovis* endocarditis would typically be less acute and is associated with underlying gastrointestinal disease (especially bowel cancer) rather than intravenous drug use.

2.42   C: Clarithromycin

Macrolides such as erythromycin and clarithromycin interfere with bacterial ribosomal function. The β-lactam agents, such as amoxicillin and glycopeptides, such as vancomycin, act by inhibiting cell wall synthesis. The fluoroquinolone ciprofloxacin inhibits bacterial DNA supercoiling by acting on DNA gyrase and topoisomerase enzymes. Trimethoprim is a diaminopyrimidine that acts by inhibiting folic acid synthesis.

2.43   A: *Listeria monocytogenes*

Neonates, the elderly and immunocompromised individuals are at increased risk of *Listeria meningitis*. Pregnant women are prone to listerial bacteraemia, but meningitis is rare; the baby rather than the mother is at risk of central nervous system infection. Amoxicillin or benzylpenicillin are the treatments of choice in listerial meningitis. Cephalosporins are not effective. The cerebrospinal fluid (CSF) findings in listerial meningitis are often only mildly abnormal. The glucose level may be normal, a lymphocytic picture may predominate and the Gram stain is often negative; partially treated meningitis of any cause could have similar CSF findings.

2.44   C: Nephritis

Cytomegalovirus (CMV) infection in HIV-positive individuals (and other immunocompromised patients) is associated with a large variety of presentations. Important manifestations include nervous system infection (retinitis, encephalitis, polyradiculopathy, myelitis), gastrointestinal disease (oesophagitis, colitis, acalculous cholecystitis, hepatitis) and pulmonary involvement (interstitial pneumonitis–much less of a problem in HIV infection than in post-transplant patients). Although urinary shedding of CMV occurs in viraemic patients, CMV nephritis has not been recognised as a significant complication of infection.

2.45   A: CCR5

The gp120, gag and gag-pol gene products and protease enzyme are all viral products rather than host derived. Gp120 is the viral ligand for the host CD4. CD8 is not involved in HIV attachment. CCR5 is now recognised to be a crucial co-receptor in the HIV replication cycle. Mutations of the gene that codes for this co-receptor have been shown to be protective against HIV infection.

2.46   E: Schistosomiasis

Schistosomiasis usually presents as a chronic disease, typically with liver (principally *Schistosoma mansoni, S. japonicum*), bowel (*S. mansoni, S. japonicum*) or urinary tract (*S. haematobium*) involvement. However, acute schistosomiasis (Katayama fever) may also occur. The clinical picture in acute schistosomiasis is dominated by allergic phenomena, including fever, urticaria, marked eosinophilia, diarrhoea, hepatosplenomegaly and wheeze. Amoebiasis and visceral leishmaniasis might explain the diarrhoea and hepatosplenomegaly respectively, but not the wheeze, urticaria and eosinophilia.

2.47   B: JC virus

This is a clinical picture suggestive of the demyelinating disease, progressive multifocal leukoencephalopathy (PML), caused by the JC virus. It typically presents over a period of weeks with focal weakness, slurring of speech, gait disturbance and changes in mental state. Patients are generally afebrile and cerebrospinal fluid (CSF) analysis is usually normal, though polymerase chain reaction (PCR) assays for JC virus may be positive. Imaging with MRI reveals focal or diffuse white matter lesions that do not enhance with contrast or display mass effect. The other pathogens listed can cause central nervous system (CNS) infection, but none fits the overall clinical scenario as well as JC virus. *Cryptococcus neoformans* and *Mycobacterium* tuberculosis would typically cause a subacute meningitis (with CSF abnormalities), while single or multiple ring-enhancing lesions are seen in cerebral toxoplasmosis. *Nocardia asteroides* is a rare cause of brain abscess in the immunocompromised.

2.48   D: Toxic shock syndrome

Not every patient who presents with vomiting and diarrhoea has gastroenteritis! The clinical picture here is a classic one for staphylococcal toxic shock syndrome (TSS). The criteria required for a diagnosis of TSS are:

- temperature ≥38.5 °C
- hypotension (systolic blood pressure < 90 mmHg)
- rash with subsequent desquamation, particularly on palms and soles
- involvement of at least three of the following organ/systems:
    - gastrointestinal (diarrhoea, vomiting)
    - musculoskeletal (severe myalgia or raised CPK)
    - mucous membranes (hyperaemia of conjunctivae, pharynx or vagina)

- renal (renal impairment)
- hepatic (abnormal liver function tests)
- thrombocytopenia
- CNS (disorientation without focal neurology)
- other conditions must also be excluded (eg measles).

2.49   C: Genital herpes

The description is typical of genital herpes, probably HSV-2. His country of origin is irrelevant in this case. If he entered the UK recently, then 'exotic' STDs such as chancroid and LGV would need to be considered, but the clinical presentation is not suggestive of either of these. Syphilis (painless, smooth ulcers) must always be considered in genital ulcer disease, but again the clinical picture does not fit with this or with Behçet disease.

2.50   E: Toxic side-effects of isoniazid are best reduced by the concomitant use of rifabutin

Rifampicin, isoniazid, ethambutol, rifabutin and pyrazinamide are commonly used antituberculous drugs. Rifampicin and isoniazid may cause hepatitis. The toxic effects of isoniazid also include peripheral neuritis and lupus-like symptoms and can be reduced by the concomitant use of pyrazinamide. Rifabutin causes uveitis and the risk of this is raised by the concomitant use of macrolide antibiotics or triazole antifungals. The dose of rifabutin should be reduced in this situation. Capreomycin is reserved for drug-resistant cases and is associated with nephrotoxicity, ototoxicity, hepatitis and eosinophilia.

ANSWERS

Neurology

NEUROLOGY 'BEST OF FIVE' ANSWERS

3.1   A: Anterior interosseous nerve

The anterior interosseous nerve is the largest branch of the median nerve arising distal to the lateral epicondyle. It supplies flexor pollicis longus, flexor digitorum profundus to the index and sometimes middle finger and pronator quadratus. Although it accounts for less than 1% of all compression palsies in the upper limb, it is more frequently represented in MRCP Part 1 questions! The typical symptom of anterior interosseous palsy is the inability to oppose the thumb and index finger. There is inability to flex the thumb IP joint and the distal IP joint of the index finger. Pronator quadratus is also paralysed. It can be caused by both traumatic and non-traumatic aetiologies.

3.2   E: Elevated CSF protein

Guillain–Barré syndrome is an acute, often postinfective, inflammatory poly-radiculopathy presenting with ascending weakness and diminished or absent reflexes. The Miller–Fisher variant (~5% of cases) consists of ataxia, ophthal-moplegia and areflexia. During the acute phase of Guillain–Barré syndrome, cerebrospinal fluid (CSF) findings classically show an elevation in CSF protein without an elevation of white blood cells ('albuminocytological dissociation'). The CSF protein increase is thought to reflect the inflammation of local nerve roots.

3.3   C: Tremor

Valproic acid is a first-line antiepileptic drug (AED) for generalized and absence seizures and one of the most widely prescribed AEDs. However, its use of VPA may be limited by side-effects such as weight gain and postural tremor. Postural tremor has been reported to occur in between six and 45% of patients and appears to be dose dependent. The mechanism of this side-effect is not clear.

3.4   D: Perseveration

Perseveration describes a patient persisting with one course of action or pattern of behavior when a change would be appropriate and can be measured neuropsychologically with the Wisconsin Card Sort Test. At the bedside perseveration may manifest on category fluency tests ('name as many words beginning with C as possible in the next minute') as repeating words given earlier in the task or with reproduction of alternating hand sequences. It is associated with disorders of executive function and frontal lobe damage. While neglect can be caused by frontal lobe damage, it is more commonly associated with parietal damage. Hemianopia most frequently results from occipital damage; memory loss from medial temporal damage; and acalculia from parietal damage.

3.5 D: Tensilon test

Myasthenia gravis is an autoimmune disorder caused by antibodies to acetylcholine (ACh) receptors at the nerve/muscle junction. Clinically this is characterised by muscle fatiguability on repeated use that recovers following a period of rest. Bulbar muscles are most commonly (and severely) affected. The Tensilon Test involves administration of edrophonium (remember the need for a test dose and appropriate resuscitation equipment to hand) which in a positive test causes dramatic but transient improvement in muscle strength.

3.6 A: Optic neuritis

Acute visual loss and pain on eye movements (to be distinguished from headache or constant ocular pain) is of the five options most consistent with retrobulbar (optic neuritis). Ischaemic optic neuropathy causes very sudden visual loss but is typically not painful. Myasthenia gravis can cause ptosis but not acute visual loss and similarly Guillain–Barré syndrome can cause neuromuscular symptoms (Miller–Fisher variant) but not visual loss. Leber's optic atrophy develops insidiously and painlessly.

3.7 E: T1

The small muscles of the hand are supplied by fibers from the T1 nerve root that travel in the medial cord of the brachial plexus and median and ulnar nerves. Consequently the differential diagnosis of wasting of the small muscles of the hand must seek to distinguish between these different possible sites.

3.8 B: Prolactin

Posterior pituitary hormones (oxytocin, vasopression) are produced in the hypothalamus but stored and released in the posterior pituitary. Release of anterior pituitary hormones (TSH, ACTH, LH, GH, prolactin) is generally under the control of hypophysiotrophic hormones (CRH, GHRH, TRH, GnRH, SS) that promote release of their corresponding pituitary hormone, with the exception of prolactin-inhibiting hormone that inhibits secretion of prolactin.

3.9   D: Fibrillation and fasciculation potentials

Motor neurone disease is characterised by fibrillation and fasciculation visible clinically and electrophysiologically, a reduction in number and increase in amplitude of motor unit action potentials and normal excitability and conduction velocity of sensory nerve fibres. Motor conduction velocities can be in the normal range unless severely affected. Presence of conduction block is more consistent with multi-focal motor neuropathy with conduction block.

3.10   A: Elevated serum creatine kinase

Dermatomyositis is an inflammatory myopathy with characteristic cutaneous manifestations. Muscle enzyme levels are frequently abnormal in dermatomyositis and the most sensitive and specific result is an elevated creatine kinase level. Aldolase, aspartate aminotransferase (AST) and LDH levels may also be abnormal. Serum enzymes can be elevated in the absence of any clinical evidence for myositis, so can be used to monitor relapses and remissions.

3.11   B: Benign intracranial hypertension (BIH)

Despite raised intracranial pressure causing papilloedema, BIH is a condition in which consciousness is clear and there are no focal neurological signs (though 'false localising' signs, such as a sixth nerve palsy may occur). BIH often presents with headache and transient visual obscurations that presage more permanent visual failure. Computed tomography (CT) scan is normal, ie there is no hydrocephalus. Classically, BIH occurs in obese young women but can also be associated with pregnancy, the oral contraceptive pill, hypocortisolism, hypoparathyroidism, hyper- and hypovitaminosis A, tetracycline therapy and other drugs. Treatment is with weight loss, serial lumbar puncture, acetazolamide and steroids.

3.12   D: Ulnar nerve

The ulnar nerve is derived from C8 and T1 roots and in the hand innervates the hypothenar muscles, the third and fourth lumbricals, the interossei and adductor pollicis. Sensory supply is to the fifth finger, the ulnar aspect of the fourth finger and the ulnar border of the palm. The ulnar nerve may be damaged by pressure in the axilla, eg from the use of crutches, but is more commonly damaged at the elbow by trauma. Complete ulnar palsy results in a characteristic claw-hand deformity with hyperextension of the fingers at the metacarpophalangeal joints and flexion at the interphalangeal joints, most pronounced on the ulnar aspect of the hand.

Answers: Neurology

3.13   E: Normal

This is a classic history of optic neuritis. In a third of cases, there will be optic disc oedema of variable severity (and which does not correlate with either field deficit or degree of visual acuity loss), but in the majority of cases the disc appearance is normal. Disc haemorrhages are rare and pallor generally develops over the 2 months following the episode. An increase in the cup/disc ratio is a feature of glaucoma.

3.14   C: Lumbar puncture

Subarachnoid haemorrhage (SAH) has not been ruled out by the normal CT. CT is abnormal is only 80–90% of proven SAH, so when SAH is suspected a normal CT should be followed by lumbar puncture and examination of the cerebrospinal fluid (CSF) for xanthochromia.

3.15   D: Communicating hydrocephalus

Normal-pressure hydrocephalus classically presents with the triad of dementia, early onset of urinary incontinence and gait disturbance. Patients may not have all these features, but the computed tomography (CT) appearance reveals hydrocephalus with an enlarged fourth ventricle but normal or compressed cortical sulci (ie the pattern of communicating hydrocephalus). Papilloedema is not a clinical feature. Many patients improve with ventricular shunting, though cerebrospinal fluid (CSF) flow studies may identify those patients most likely to improve.

3.16   B: Right occipital lobe

Visual field defects are helpful in localising lesions. Defects restricted to one eye are likely to represent lesions to the retina or optic nerve. Bitemporal field deficits indicate a lesion of the optic chiasm. Homonymous field defects indicate pathology posterior to the chiasm. Quadrantanopia most often indicates a lesion in either the optic radiations or occipital cortex. Superior quadrantanopia indicates damage to the temporal optic radiations or inferior bank of the calcarine (primary visual) cortex. Parietal or superior calcarine lesions will, in contrast, produce an inferior quadrantanopia. Hemianopia typically results from damage to both banks of the calcarine cortex, ie a contralateral occipital lesion.

3.17   C: Brown-Séquard syndrome

This question tests knowledge of spinal cord anatomy, specifically the distinction between crossed and uncrossed sensory pathways. In the spinal cord, fibres carrying vibration and joint-position sense ascend ipsilaterally to the cuneate and gracilis nuclei in the brainstem, where they decussate and ultimately project to contralateral primary sensory cortex in the postcentral gyrus. In contrast, pain and temperature fibres ascend contralaterally in the spinothalamic tracts. So, cord hemisection (eg Brown-Séquard syndrome, most commonly associated with multiple sclerosis) can lead to ipsilateral loss of proprioception but contralateral loss of pain sensation. Motor function is lost ipsilaterally in cord hemisection due to interruption of descending cortico-spinal fibres.

3.18   C: Right abducens

The way in which oculomotor mononeuropathies affect diplopia can be predicted with three rules. First, paresis of horizontally acting muscles causes predominantly horizontal diplopia and of vertical muscles predominantly causes vertical diplopia. Second, the direction in which the separation of the two images is maximal is the direction of action of the weak muscle. Finally, covering the affected eye leads to disappearance of the outer (false) image. In this case, these suggest right lateral rectus palsy.

3.19   D: Sensitivity

The sensitivity of a test for a particular disease refers to how good that test is at correctly identifying people who have that disease. It represents the probability that the test will produce a true positive result when used on an infected population (as compared to a reference or 'gold standard'). A test with high sensitivity will have few false negatives. The specificity of a test, on the other hand, is concerned with how good the test is at correctly identifying people who are well and do not have a disease. A test with high specificity will have few false positives. The positive predictive value of a test is the probability that a person is infected when a positive test result is observed. On the other hand, the negative predictive value of a test is the probability that a person is not infected when a negative test result is observed. Sensitivity and specificity are both measures of the accuracy of a diagnostic test.

3.20   A: Carbamazepine

This history is typical of trigeminal neuralgia. This is a disorder of the fifth cranial (trigeminal) nerve that causes episodes of intense, stabbing, electric shock-like pain in the distribution of the trigeminal nerve (most frequently, in the maxillary and mandibular divisions). Initial treatment is usually with anti-convulsant drugs, though antidepressants may be helpful. If medication is ineffective or not tolerated, neurosurgical procedures may be required.

3.21 C: Posterior inferior cerebellar artery occlusion

This individual has suffered damage to the lateral medulla, resulting in Wallen-berg syndrome. Wallenberg syndrome comprises vertigo, nausea, vomiting, ipsilateral cerebellar signs, contralateral sensory disturbance on the body, saccadic abnormalities, dysphagia, dysphonia, dysarthria and a Horner syn-drome. The syndrome is most commonly caused by occlusion of the posterior inferior cerebellar artery or one of its branches supplying the lower brainstem.

3.22 C: Intravenous phenytoin 15 mg/kg

This is established status epilepticus and initial treatment with intravenous lorazepam has not worked. It would not be appropriate to give diazepam (lorazepam and diazepam are equally effective in terminating status but have the same mechanism of action) or a lower dose of lorazepam. In this situation, the best drug to give would be an intravenous infusion of phenytoin at a dose of 15–18 mg/kg. Phenobarbital (phenobarbitone) could also be used, but the typical dosage is 10 mg/kg.

3.23 B: Creutzfeldt–Jakob disease (CJD)

Sporadic CJD predominantly affects late-middle-aged individuals with a mean age at death in the late 60s. Memory impairment and cerebellar ataxia are common early features. Subsequently, rapidly progressive dementia, ataxia and myoclonus are common features. The median duration of illness is four months and about 65% of cases die within 6 months.

3.24 E: No driving for 1 year

Medical aspects of fitness to drive in the United Kingdom are described in full at http://www.dvla.gov.uk/at_a_glance/content.htm. For a single unprovoked seizure, the regulations state that the patient will lose their licence to drive a private motor vehicle (Group 1) for 1 year and will require a medical review before restarting driving.

3.25   E: Propranolol

Prophylactic therapy should be considered in migraine when acute therapy alone is failing to control the symptoms, typically when patients experience more than three or four attacks per month. A variety of agents can be tried, but the most common are α-blockers, amitriptyline and other antidepressants, calcium-channel blockers and anticonvulsants.

3.26   C: Anti-Yo antibodies

Paraneoplastic syndromes are immune-mediated syndromes associated with particular cancers. There are several different CNS-associated paraneoplastic syndromes, but the ataxia here suggests paraneoplastic cerebellar degeneration in the absence of any cerebellar metastases. This occurs most frequently in breast and ovarian malignancy and is associated with anti-Yo antibodies. Treatment of the underlying malignancy may prevent progression of symptoms, but frequently does not result in improvement. Anti-Hu antibodies are often seen in subacute sensorimotor neuropathies associated with small-cell lung cancer. Anti-Ro antibodies are seen in Sjögren syndrome, systemic lupus erythematosus (SLE) and other rheumatological syndromes. Acetylcholine receptor antibodies are characteristic of myasthenia gravis. Finally, calcium-channel antibodies are seen in Eaton–Lambert myasthenic syndrome.

3.27   D: Optic neuritis

Optic neuritis typically presents with loss of vision, abnormal colour vision and eye pain. The initial attack is unilateral in about 75% of adult patients and the mean age of onset is in the third decade.

3.28   C: Toxoplasmosis

Toxoplasmosis is the most frequent cause of intracranial mass lesions in AIDS, causing single or multiple brain abscesses. Clinically, the presentation is heterogeneous, ranging from a febrile illness to focal neurological deficits, developing either subacutely or acutely. Small to medium size ring-enhancing lesions with surrounding oedema on computed tomography (CT) suggest the diagnosis.

3.29   C: Carbamazepine

This is a description of simple partial seizures, specifically a focal motor seizure. This would be best treated with carbamazepine, although phenytoin would also be a possibility. Levetiracetam and vigabatrin are primarily used for adjunctive treatment of partial seizures; lorazepam is used in the acute treatment of status epilepticus.

3.30 B: Partially treated bacterial meningitis

This is a typical presentation of partially treated bacterial meningitis. All of the other options should reduce glucose levels.

3.31 A: Shy–Drager syndrome

The combination of parkinsonism (tremor, rigidity and bradykinesia) with symptoms suggestive of autonomic failure suggest multiple system atrophy, also called Shy–Drager syndrome. Other autonomic symptoms may include sweating abnormalities, gastrointestinal disturbance, abnormal Valsalva response, difficulty with urination or sexual function and loss of the normal beat-to-beat variability in heart rate.

3.32 C: Multiple system atrophy

All of these diagnoses can be associated with extrapyramidal signs. Typically, the triad of rigidity, resting tremor and bradykinesia is associated with Parkinson disease. Here, the presence of additional autonomic symptoms and signs suggests a 'Parkinson's plus' syndrome. Postural hypotension may occur in patients with Parkinson disease, but is typically mild and secondary to (levodopa) medication. Multiple system atrophy represents a group of disorders combining parkinsonism with moderate to severe autonomic neuropathy. In this group of disorders, the parkinsonism is typically poorly responsive to treatment.

3.33 C: Right abducens nerve

Three cranial nerves control the upper eyelid, eye movements and pupils, the oculomotor (third), trochlear (fourth) and abducens (sixth). Horizontal diplopia implies a weakness of the horizontally acting muscles, vertical diplopia the vertically acting muscles. Diplopia is maximal in the direction of action of the weak muscle and when the eye to which the weak muscle belongs is covered, then the outer (false) image is obscured. So, in this case, the diplopia is caused by a weak right lateral rectus, so indicating right abducens palsy. This is most likely to have been caused by poorly controlled diabetes mellitus.

3.34   E: Temporal lobe uncus across the tentorium

Space-occupying lesions can impair consciousness either through direct exten-sion of the lesion into the mid-brain and brainstem or, more commonly, by lateral and downward displacement of these structures with or without hernia-tion of the medial part of the temporal lobe through the tentorium. This lateral displacement typically crushes the upper mid-brain against the opposite free edge of the tentorium, causing an upgoing plantar ipsilateral to the hemispheric lesions. All forms of brainstem herniation can cause depression of respiration, extensor posturing and bilateral upgoing plantars. The uncal syndrome differs mainly in that early drowsiness is accompanied or preceded by unilateral pupillary dilatation,often (but not always) due to compression of the oculomo-tor nerve by the herniated uncus.

3.35   C: Posterior inferior cerebellar artery

Ipsilateral Horner syndrome and contralateral loss of pain and temperature sensation indicate damage in the dorsolateral region of the medulla, known as Wallenberg syndrome. Lower vestibular nuclei are often involved, resulting in vertigo, vomiting and nystagmus; involvement of the inferior cerebellar pedun-cle will result in ipsilateral limb ataxia. This medullary syndrome is most often caused by occlusion of the posterior inferior cerebellar artery, although in some cases an occlusion of the parent vertebral artery can be responsible.

3.36   A: Acoustic neuroma

A cerebellopontine angle lesion is indicated by the combination of absent corneal reflex and sensorineural deafness. No other single central lesion could account for these signs. Lesions arising in the pons, such as multiple sclerosis or brainstem astrocytoma, are likely to present with more complex neuro-logical signs. Similarly, extrinsic lesions, such as basilar artery aneurysm or nasopharyngeal carcinoma, are more likely to present with isolated single compressive cranial nerve lesions.

3.37   C: Left thalamic metastasis

The dense sensory impairment described here is typical for a space-occupying thalamic lesion and the progressive history over several months makes meta-stasis more likely than either demyelination or stroke. Sensory loss caused by a cortical lesion is rarely complete.

3.38   A: Craniopharyngioma

Craniopharyngiomas compress the optic chiasm from above and behind, producing a bitemporal hemianopia that spreads up from the lower fields into the upper fields. In adults, pituitary dysfunction secondary to craniopharyngioma is variable, but the tumour may block the third ventricle causing hydrocephalus and dementia. Pituitary macroadenomas cause a bitemporal hemianopia, which typically spreads down from the upper fields as the optic chiasm is damaged from below.

3.39   A: Common peroneal nerve

The common peroneal nerve is most often damaged by compression at the fibula neck, where it winds around the bone. The nerve is motor to tibialis anterior and the peronei, causing weakness of dorsiflexion and eversion respectively. As nerve roots L5 and S1 control these movements, differentiation from an L5 root lesion requires demonstration of intact eversion in the presence of severe weakness of dorsiflexion. The common peroneal nerve is sensory to a small patch of skin on the dorsum of the foot between the big and second toes, but often there is little or no sensory loss detectable clinically.

3.40   C: Meningococcal meningitis

This patient has an acute bacterial meningitis and is predisposed to infection due to his splenectomy. Meningococcal meningitis is the most likely diagnosis, due to the characteristic petechiae and purpura. Although these skin manifestations can also be seen occasionally with *Haemophilus* and pneumococcal meningitis, they are much more common in meningococcal meningitis.

3.41   D: Episodic memory deficit

The gradual development of forgetfulness is the major symptom of Alzheimer's disease and is characterised on neuropsychological testing by a deficit of episodic memory. Other failures of cortical function, including all the disorders here, may be manifest but typically occur later in the course of the disease. Visual hallucinations are often a prominent feature of a less common form of dementia, corticobasal degeneration; and frontal syndromes, such as disinhibition, together with progressive language impairment, are seen in Pick disease.

3.42 A: Huntington disease

Progressive chorea, emotional disturbance and dementia with onset in the fourth decade are typical of Huntington disease. Patients may lack or conceal a family history; diagnosis is usually easy, as the mutation (CAG repeat expansion in the Huntington gene) has been identified. The other diagnoses listed here can cause an extrapyramidal movement disorder, but choreiform movements are less common and/or prominent and intellectual decline is not typically a presenting feature.

3.43 C: Left parietal lobe

This woman has a partial Gerstmann syndrome, affecting the dominant (left) parietal lobe. The characteristic features are inability to name the fingers of the two hands (finger agnosia), confusion of left and right sides of the body, inability to calculate (dyscalculia) or write (dysgraphia). Damage to the superior part of the optic radiation in the underlying white matter causes a contralateral homonymous lower quadrantanopia (in contrast to the homonymous superior quadrantanopia following temporal lesions). Often the patient will be unaware of the visual field deficit.

3.44 D: Haem

Severe symmetrical polyneuropathy, together with abdominal pain and neuropsychiatric symptoms (or confusion), is typical of acute intermittent porphyria. This is a disorder of haem metabolism inherited as an autosomal dominant syndrome, with attacks often precipitated by drugs such as oestrogens, phenytoin and sulphonamides. The neuropathy often involves the motor nerves more severely than the sensory; symptoms may begin in the arms or legs, usually distally but occasionally also in the proximal limb girdle.

3.45 B: Guillain–Barré syndrome

Guillain–Barré syndrome (GBS) is an acute ascending polyneuropathy; as here, sensory symptoms are typically out of proportion to the weakness. Areflexia is characteristic and progression can be rapid with respiratory failure and death. The immediate diagnostic problem is to differentiate GBS from acute spinal cord compression (which would produce an upper motor neurone lesion in the legs with hyper-reflexia and upgoing plantars and does not produce facial weakness). Cerebrospinal fluid (CSF) is typically acellular or shows a mild lymphocytosis, but with a grossly elevated protein.

3.46   A: Carbamazepine

This woman has complex partial seizures, with a typical aura followed by loss of consciousness and subsequent post-ictal confusion. While unconscious during the fit, her behaviour shows automatisms and semipurposive features. Carbamazepine is the drug of choice for complex partial seizures or sometimes sodium valproate. Phenytoin can be successful but can also sometimes worsen complex partial seizures. Lamotrigine, vigabatrin and gabapentin are also useful, but only as second-line agents.

3.47   E: Sagittal sinus

Parasagittal biparietal or bifrontal haemorrhagic infarctions are common sequelae of sagittal sinus thrombosis. Oral contraceptives, the immediate post-partum period, hypercoagulable states and dehydration all predispose to sagittal sinus thrombosis. The presence of multiple lesions that are not in typical arterial territories and the prominent epileptic fits, favour this diagnosis.

3.48   E: Vitamin B$_{12}$

Subacute combined degeneration of the spinal cord, due to vitamin B$_{12}$ deficiency, results in degeneration of the posterior columns (vibration and joint-position sense), followed by progressive development of upper motor neurone signs in the legs. Spinal cord involvement is roughly symmetrical, but can progress to dementia and visual impairment due to optic neuropathy. Thiamine deficiency may give rise to Wernicke syndrome (ophthalmoplegia, ataxia and confusion) or to beriberi (peripheral neuropathy). Pyridoxine deficiency gives rise to a chronic painful sensorimotor neuropathy. This can be caused by administration of isoniazid (for tuberculosis), which increases the excretion of pyridoxine; hence isoniazid is always administered in conjunction with pyridoxine.

3.49   D: Radial

The radial nerve in the axilla is often damaged by the incorrect use of a crutch, which causes weakness of all the radial nerve-innervated muscles. In addition to triceps and the wrist and finger extensors, there is also weakness of brachioradialis. Triceps is only variably involved, for reasons that are unclear.

3.50   B: Creutzfeldt–Jakob disease

This is a rapidly progressive and severe dementia associated with cerebellar ataxia, diffuse myoclonic jerks and other neurological abnormalities. Myoclonus is typical and progressive, even during the later stages when the patient is stuporous or comatose. The disease is invariably fatal, usually within a few months. The electroencephalogram (EEG) pattern is characteristic but diagnosis relies on either specialised tests for prion protein in CSF or direct brain biopsy.

ANSWERS

Psychiatry

PSYCHIATRY 'BEST OF FIVE' ANSWERS

4.1   E: Cerebral involvement is an indicator of poor prognosis

CNS involvement occurs in about a third of cases of systemic lupus erythematosus (SLE). Psychiatric symptoms occur in 60% of cases: the excess is due to both psychological reactions to illness and corticosteroid side-effects. The most common presentations are acute organic states and neurotic disorders; schizophrenia-like syndromes are rare. Mental symptoms are seldom the first signs of SLE (which are usually fever, malaise and arthralgia). When present, psychiatric symptoms often fluctuate, usually remit within 6 weeks, but may recur. The presence of cerebral vasculitis substantially worsens prognosis.

4.2   D: It is associated with reduced life expectancy in severe schizophrenia

Tardive dyskinesia is characterised by chewing, sucking and grimacing of the face and choreoathetoid movements. It occurs in about one-fifth of patients receiving long-term treatment with neuroleptic medication such as phenothiazines or butyrophenones. Increased incidence is seen in women and with increasing age but not with brain damage or previous treatment with ECT. Few treatments are helpful and stopping the offending drug may produce paradoxical worsening. There is decreased life expectancy when functional psychosis and severe dyskinesia are both present.

4.3   C: Clouding of consciousness

Puerperal psychosis is not thought to be a distinct form of mental illness. It has a number of features in common with post-operative psychoses, including acute confusion and therefore clouding of consciousness. The disorder can present with features similar to an affective or schizophreniform psychosis. Clinical features may therefore include labile mood, overactivity, hallucinations and delusions. Onset is most commonly between two and fourteen days after parturition. A history of mental illness may be present, but making a diagnosis depends more on the presence of active symptoms at the time of assessment.

4.4   A: Says he does not know the answers and cannot do the tests

People with most forms of dementia tend to lack insight into their problems and attempt testing willingly but do poorly at tasks. Low mood and personality changes are less helpful diagnostically because they can be associated with depression or early dementia, as can subjective short-term memory loss.

4.5   B: ECT can cause short-term memory loss

Randomised controlled trials have compared ECT to 'sham' ECT (the application of a general anaesthetic and muscle relaxant but no subsequent ECT). ECT is superior to sham ECT in the treatment of severe depression. Antidepressants are also useful in the treatment of severe depression, but ECT produces quicker results. Therefore, in potentially life-threatening situations, ECT is the treatment of choice. ECT results in brief memory disturbances after each treatment. There is less conclusive evidence that it causes any long-term cognitive impairment. As muscle relaxants are used, patients do not convulse in an uncontrolled manner.

4.6   C: Improvement of mood every evening

Antidepressants are most effective when a patient has evidence of clinical depression. Clinical features include: persistent depressed mood accompanied by guilt or worthlessness; persistent low levels of concentration, energy, appetite and libido; early-morning wakening and diurnal variation of mood, with depression being consistently worse in the morning. The presence of these symptoms suggests an underlying chemical imbalance that can respond to antidepressants.

4.7   B: There is an accompanying sense of impending doom

Panic disorder consists of unpredictable attacks of severe anxiety. Attacks include somatic and psychological symptoms. The latter include a fear that something drastic is about to happen, such as collapse or death. As a consequence, patients often try to escape hurriedly the situation they are in. The attacks last between a few minutes and half an hour and are rarely longer in duration. Continuous feelings of nervousness are more typical of generalised anxiety disorder.

4.8   A: Abnormal psychomotor activity

Delirium is an acute-onset syndrome characterised by inattention and an impaired level of consciousness. Thinking is often disorganised and perseverative. Perceptual disturbances include misinterpretations, illusions and hallucinations. There is disturbance of the sleep–wake cycle, with insomnia and daytime sleepiness. Psychomotor activity may be increased or decreased. Disorientation and memory impairment are common. The patient has no insight during episodes of confusion and amnesia for the episode once it has resolved. 'Catastrophic reaction' has been described in dementing patients, which is characterised by marked agitation secondary to the subjective awareness of intellectual deficits under stressful circumstances.

4.9   E: Visual hallucinations

The core diagnostic features of Lewy body dementia are: fluctuating cognition with pronounced variations in attention and alertness, recurrent complex visual hallucinations and spontaneous features of parkinsonism. Features A to D are *supportive* features including 'confusing dreams with reality', which is caused by rapid eye movement (REM) sleep behavioural disorder. Postural hypotension is caused by general autonomic instability and about 50% of people with Lewy body dementia will be sensitive to the side-effects of neuroleptics, which exacerbate parkinsonian symptoms and may hasten cognitive decline and death.

4.10   C: Korsakoff syndrome

The key features of this are both retrograde (loss of memory for events before the onset of the illness) and anterograde amnesia (inability to lay down new memories). Gaps in memory are filled in by confabulation (the unconscious production of false memories). These symptoms are persistent (unlike the fluctuating condition of delirium) and procedural memory and procedural daily living skills are intact (unlike in Alzheimer disease). Alcoholic hallucinosis is not associated with confusion and occurs in clear consciousness.

4.11   D: Nystagmus

The 'classic triad' of Wernicke syndrome (nystagmus, ataxia and external ophthalmoplegia) may not be present. Ocular signs are found in 95% and nystagmus is the most common, followed by ophthalmoplegia and conjugate gaze palsy. Ataxia occurs in approximately 80% and peripheral neuropathy in 20%. MRI changes may be suggestive of Wernicke's but have low sensitivity (around 50%). Anterograde amnesia is characteristic of Korsakoff disease.

4.12   B: A denial that she is underweight

Anorexia nervosa is characterised by deliberate self-induced weight loss. Key features include body image distortion, with underweight patients believing they are fat. As a consequence of self-induced weight loss, there are endocrine abnormalities that result in amenorrhoea. Her BMI is less than 17.5 kg/m^2, the lower limit for post-pubertal women. However, the BMI is less important as a diagnostic factor than the abnormal psychopathology described above.

4.13   A: Chlordiazepoxide

Clozapine and haloperidol are antipsychotics. Procyclidine is an anticholinergic drug that is often prescribed to individuals who develop extrapyramidal side effects from antipsychotics. Sodium valproate is prescribed less often, but has been indicated for individuals with prominent affective components to their schizophrenic illness. Chlordiazepoxide is a benzodiazepine used in alcohol detoxification.

4.14   A: Anorgasmia

SSRIs are effective antidepressants with a less sedative effect than tricyclics, few antimuscarinic effects and low cardiotoxicity. The most frequent side-effects are gastrointestinal (diarrhoea, nausea and vomiting), which are dose-related. Restlessness, anxiety, insomnia and sweating may be marked initially. Side-effects also include anorexia, weight loss and allergic reactions, including anaphylaxis (all more common with fluoxetine), convulsions (particularly with fluvoxamine), extrapyramidal reactions and a withdrawal syndrome (particularly with paroxetine), abnormalities of hepatic enzymes (particularly with fluvoxamine and sertraline) and sexual dysfunction, including anorgasmia and ejaculatory failure in men (particularly with paroxetine and fluoxetine). Suicidal ideation has been associated with SSRIs but causality has not been established.

4.15   B: Dysthymic disorder

This is chronic low mood that does not fulfil the criteria for recurrent depressive disorder in terms of either severity or duration of episodes. Sufferers usually have periods of days or weeks when they describe themselves as unwell, but most of the time (often for months at a time) they have low mood that only mildly interferes with day-to-day functioning. This has also been known as dysthymic personality disorder.

4.16   E: Cyclothymia

This is a persistent instability of mood involving numerous periods of depression and mild elation, none of which is sufficiently severe or prolonged to justify a diagnosis of bipolar affective disorder or recurrent depressive disorder. Because the mood swings are relatively mild and the periods of mood elevation may be enjoyable, cyclothymia frequently fails to come to medical attention. This disorder is frequently found in the relatives of patients with bipolar affective disorder. Some patients with cyclothymia eventually develop bipolar affective disorder.

4.17 B: Caudate atrophy

The patient may not be aware of a family history for a number of reasons, including estrangement from family or intellectual deterioration. Huntington disease is an uncommon autosomal dominant disorder affecting four to seven people per 100 000 of the population. Senile and drug-induced choreas are much more frequently encountered. Anatomically, the frontal lobes and the caudate nucleus are most severely affected by neuronal loss and gliosis. Ventricular dilatation does occur in Huntington disease but is less specific than the finding of caudate atrophy.

4.18 A: Alzheimer dementia

Individuals with mental retardation are at a higher risk of developing a number of mental illnesses, such as schizophrenia or a mood disorder. Epilepsy is found in over 10% of those with Down syndrome aged over 40. Alzheimer dementia is found in approximately 95% of individuals with Down syndrome aged over 40.

4.19 C: Quetiapine

Typical antipsychotics all have some D_2 antagonist activity and can so produce parkinsonian side-effects. Sulpiride acts exclusively on D_2 receptors. Haloperidol acts at a number of receptor sites, but is a potent D_2 antagonist. Chlorpromazine acts as a weaker D_2 antagonist. All atypical antipsychotics have a much lower propensity to produce parkinsonian side-effects. However, at high doses risperidone can produce extrapyramidal side-effects.

4.20 A: Autochthonous delusions

Psychosis is defined as the presence of delusions, hallucinations or specific abnormalities of behaviour, such as catatonia, severe psychomotor retardation or overactivity. Autochthonous (primary) delusions are first-rank symptoms of schizophrenia. Hallucinations of any modality are a feature of psychosis. Hypnagogical and hypnapompic hallucinations are exceptions as they refer to auditory hallucinations experienced not in clear consciousness, but respectively as one drifts into sleep or awakens. Echopraxia is a feature of cognitive impairment. Tardive dyskinesia may be a result of long-term antipsychotic medication, but does not indicate current psychosis.

Answers: Psychiatry

4.21   B: Catalepsy

Catatonia is a disorder of motor activity and can occur in schizophrenia. Catalepsy, also known as 'waxy' flexibility, is a disorder of muscle tone, which can result in patients maintaining what are often very uncomfortable postures for long periods of time without moving. Stupor, excitement and negativism are other features of catatonia. Cataplexy is the sudden loss of muscle tone. Stereotypes are repeated non-goal-directed movements, eg rocking back and forth. Mannerisms are goal-directed movements that occur out of context.

4.22   C: Prognathism

Fragile-X syndrome is the second commonest cause of mental retardation in males. Clinical features include macro-orchidism and facial abnormalities, such as prognathism and hypertelorism. A single palmar crease can occur in fragile-X but also occurs in Down syndrome. Strabismus occurs more frequently with Down syndrome. Learning difficulties accompanied by an absence of male secondary sexual characteristics is associated with Klinefelter syndrome. Tall stature is more commonly associated with XYY sex chromosome abnormalities.

4.23   C: He has apraxia on bedside testing

Dementia affects 1:5 of those over 80, so family history is less indicative in older people. Depression can occur in the early stages of Alzheimer disease but is not characteristic. Incontinence and abnormal gait occur in the later stages of Alzheimer's. Apraxia is a characteristic symptom of Alzheimer's and occurs with the other signs such as impaired episodic memory and functional impairment.

4.24   C: The presence of secondary gain

Munchausen syndrome is a factitious disorder. This disorder is defined as the voluntary production of physical or psychological symptoms, which can be attributed to a need to adopt the sick role. Secondary gain is defined as the presence of an advantage gained as a result of having symptoms – in this case attention and admission. Munchausen syndrome specifically differs from malingering in that there is no fraudulent simulation of symptoms. Financial gain is therefore not a motive. Alcohol dependence may be present but is not particularly associated with the syndrome. Simulated psychiatric symptoms are common, such as 'hearing voices.' Hearing voices inside one's head is a pseudohallucination and therefore not a true psychotic phenomenon. Voices heard outside one's head are more characteristic of a genuine hallucination.

4.25   E: Bradycardia

Neuroleptic malignant syndrome is a rare but potentially life-threatening complication of neuroleptic therapy. It consists of mental state changes, including confusion and mutism, as well as physical abnormalities. Autonomic dysfunction, including elevated or labile blood pressure, tachycardia, pyrexia and diaphoresis can occur, as well as dysphagia, tremor and incontinence. Treatment varies, depending on the severity of presentation, but always includes the cessation of antipsychotic therapy.

4.26   E: Increased plasma amylase

Hypokalaemia occurs secondary to self-induced vomiting. Hypercholesterolaemia is thought to occur via complex mechanism mediated by low lipid intake, hypoglycemia and hypoinsulinemia. Anorexia nervosa is associated with relative lymphocytosis and increased growth hormone levels.

4.27   C: Primary delusion

All of the options listed are features of schizophrenia. A delusion is a false, unshakeable belief out of keeping with a patient's social and cultural background. Primary delusions appear suddenly and with full conviction. Delusional perceptions are examples of primary delusions and are of first-rank importance in the diagnosis of schizophrenia. A delusional perception occurs when an individual forms an instantaneous delusion after a normal perception, for example suddenly believing you are Jesus on seeing a blue car drive past. A secondary delusion is derived from an abnormal mental phenomenon, for example believing oneself to be Jesus because the hallucinatory voice of God has told you so. Other first-rank symptoms are audible thoughts, third-person auditory hallucinations, passivity and thought broadcasting, insertion or withdrawal.

4.28   C: Second person auditory hallucinations

These also occur in depression or mania. Auditory hallucinations included in Schneider's 'first-rank' symptoms of schizophrenia are: hearing thoughts spoken aloud, hearing voices referring to himself/herself (third person) and auditory hallucinations in the form of a running commentary. A, B and D are also 'first-rank' symptoms.

4.29   A: Cognitive behavioural therapy

The patient described has features of clinical depression. Key diagnostic features are depressed mood, increased fatiguability and anhedonia (loss of interest and enjoyment). Trials of different kinds of psychotherapy are difficult to conduct. However, for cases of mild-to-moderate depression, cognitive behavioural therapy (CBT) has been shown to be as effective as antidepressants.

4.30   B: Florid affective symptoms

Prominent mood (affective) symptoms are associated with better prognosis. Indicators of poor prognosis in schizophrenia include insidious onset, long duration of first illness, emotional blunting, social withdrawal, high expressed emotion among the family, poor psychosexual functioning and soft neurological signs.

4.31   E: Thought alienation

Thought alienation is a disorder of the possession of thought. The individual has the experience that his thoughts are under the control of an outside person or force. Examples of thought alienation include thought withdrawal, thought insertion and thought broadcasting. Hallucinations are perceptions experienced without any external stimulus. Hallucinations heard when going to sleep (hypnagogic) or on waking (hypnapompic) can occur in tired, healthy people and in sleep disorders such as narcolepsy. Depersonalisation occurs when a person feels numb and unreal. Derealisation occurs when his environment feels unreal. Both states are unpleasant and occur in a large number of psychiatric disorders, especially anxiety states, depression and schizophrenia. They can also occur in tired, healthy individuals.

4.32   A: Amphetamine

Amphetamines can produce a schizophrenia-like illness in otherwise healthy individuals. Cannabis is thought to bring on schizophrenia early in susceptible individuals, but is otherwise unlikely to produce a schizophreniform psychosis. LSD and psilocybin (found in magic mushrooms) produce perceptual abnormalities, mainly during intoxication, but do not produce first-rank schizophrenic symptoms. Heroin use does not produce psychotic symptoms.

4.33   A: Inability to feel sadness

Uncomplicated grief reactions consist of three stages. The first stage should only last a maximum of a few days and is characterised by denial and numbness. The second stage can last up to 6 months or 1 year. This stage is characterised by intense sadness, loneliness, yearning for the dead person, anorexia, poor sleep and anxiety. Fleeting hallucinations of the dead person may also occur. In the third stage, symptoms subside and there is gradual acceptance and readjustment. Pathological grief consists of a delayed, inhibited or abnormally long period of grieving. There may also be a typical depressive picture with marked feelings of worthlessness, psychomotor retardation or functional impairment.

4.34   D: Intrusive flashbacks

Repeated reliving of trauma through flashbacks (intrusive memories) or nightmares is typical, with avoidance of situations that might trigger painful memories. The traumatic event must be exceptionally violent or catastrophic in nature. There is often accompanying autonomic hyperarousal, emotional blunting, anhedonia and other features of anxiety and depression, but these are not essential to make the diagnosis. Believing his attackers have followed him to the UK is suggestive of a persecutory delusion, which is not typical of PTSD.

4.35   B: Thioridazine

Antipsychotic drugs cause QTc lengthening in a dose-related manner. This is most commonly associated with thioridazine followed by droperidol. This confers an increased risk of drug-induced arrhythmia, most commonly prolonged QTc precedes torsade de pointes.

4.36   E: Somatisation disorder

Somatisation disorder is characterised by multiple, changing physical symptoms that have been present for at least 2 years. As a result of the symptoms, the patient's life becomes considerably disrupted. However, the patient refuses to accept reassurance from negative test results and medical opinion. In hypochondriacal disorder the patient's focus is not on the symptoms, but on the presence of an underlying serious disease such as cancer or cardiovascular disease. The terms dissociative (psychiatric) and conversion (physical) disorder have replaced the old-fashioned and imprecise term 'hysteria'.

4.37   A: Acute onset

Dementia has an insidious and chronic course and patients may have neuro-logical signs, abnormal electroencephalogram (EEG) (non-specific changes) and a persistently poor performance on cognitive testing. In depressive pseudo-dementia there tends to be a more acute onset and performance may improve during the day as diurnal mood variation leads to improvements in attention and concentration.

4.38   E: Negativism

Schizophrenic symptoms can be divided into positive and negative. Positive symptoms often occur in acute episodes and include hallucinations, delusions, formal thought disorder and bizarre behaviour. Negative symptoms are asso-ciated with a more chronic picture and may be very disabling. These symptoms include poverty of speech (alogia), poor motivation and initiative (avolition), an inability to derive pleasure from activities (anhedonia), emotional blunting and attentional deficits. Catatonia can occur in schizophrenia and is a disorder of psychomotor activity. Symptoms include stupor, excitement, waxy flexibility, mutism and negativism.

4.39   C: Perseverating responses

Frontal lobe dysfunction can result in personality changes, disinhibition and euphoria or apathy and slowing of thought and motor activity. Perseveration of actions and difficulties in planning and executing actions can also occur. Impaired 5-minute recall can suggest bilateral temporal lobe dysfunction. Sensory dysphasia can occur if the dominant temporal lobe is affected. Right–left disorientation is part of Gerstmann syndrome, affecting the dominant parietal lobe. Hypersomnia may result from dysfunction of the diencephalon and brainstem.

4.40   D: Intramuscular lorazepam

In a patient who is neuroleptic-naïve, antipsychotics should be administered with caution. Parenteral administration should be avoided if possible until the response to an oral dose has been assessed. Reasons include an increased risk of cardiovascular complications when antipsychotics are administered parent-erally to highly agitated individuals. There is also the risk of acute dystonic reactions. Chlorpromazine, in addition, is irritant when administered intramus-cularly. Benzodiazepines, often followed by oral antipsychotics, are generally a safer option in this situation. Intramuscular diazepam, however, is poorly absorbed.

4.41   A: Acknowledging that this belief is irrational, but still refusing

Obsessional thoughts often involve contamination as a theme. They may involve an accompanying compulsive act or ritual that lessens the anxiety associated with the thought. The ritual itself is not inherently pleasurable. Obsessional thoughts must be recognised as the individual's own thoughts and are therefore not part of a psychotic process. The thoughts are commonly perceived as being senseless and are resisted, but at a cost of considerable anxiety.

4.42   E: Short-term memory loss

All of the sequelae listed can occur after a head injury. However, short-term memory loss is usually the most persistent cognitive dysfunction. Focal brain pathology after a head injury can result in focal deficits. For example, executive dysfunction, including impaired planning and executing of actions, can occur with frontal lobe pathology.

4.43   A: Ataxia

The answer to this question is ataxia as you have been asked which abnormality is most likely to indicate toxicity. Tremor can occur at therapeutic plasma levels, whereas ataxia should only occur in toxicity. Lithium has a low therapeutic index, but can produce a number of unpleasant side-effects at therapeutic levels (0.4–1.1 mmol/l). These include fine tremor, nausea, vomiting, diarrhoea and metallic taste. A coarse tremor, ataxia, slurred speech, disorientation and convulsions can occur in toxicity.

4.44   C: Fasciculations

Conversion disorders frequently present to doctors. They are characterised by the presence of symptoms or deficits involving voluntary motor or sensory functions. In motor conversion disorders, the patient may not be able to contract a particular muscle group. However, tests often show that the muscles are able to contract when the patient's attention is diverted. Changes in reflexes are not present, but disuse atrophy can occur in chronic cases.

4.45   E: The majority of cases are preceded by anorexia nervosa

To make a diagnosis of bulimia nervosa there must be recurrent episodes of binge eating – eating larger than normal amounts of food, accompanied by a loss of control over eating. In addition there must be recurrent compensatory behaviour to prevent weight gain, eg self-induced vomiting, laxative or diuretic abuse, fasting or excessive exercising. A fear of fatness is also prominent. About one-third of patients with bulimia may previously have had anorexia nervosa. If all features are present apart from compensatory behaviour, the condition is known as binge-eating disorder.

REVISION CHECKLISTS

BASIC SCIENCES: REVISION CHECKLIST

Physiology
- ☐ Changes in pregnancy
- ☐ Haemoglobin function
- ☐ Physiology of bone
- ☐ Aetiology of oedema
- ☐ Magnesium
- ☐ Exercise

Pathology
- ☐ Amyloid plaques

Hormone and mediator biochemistry
- ☐ Atrial natriuretic peptides
- ☐ Insulin/insulin resistance
- ☐ Adenosine
- ☐ ADH
- ☐ Aldosterone

- ☐ Angiotensin/Renin
- ☐ EDRF (nitric oxide)
- ☐ H2 receptors
- ☐ Neurotransmitters
- ☐ Prostacyclin
- ☐ Somatostatin
- ☐ Steroid receptors

Miscellaneous
- ☐ Apolipoproteins
- ☐ Alpha1-antitrypsin
- ☐ Mitochondrial DNA function
- ☐ Oncogenes/Tumour suppressor genes
- ☐ Statistics
- ☐ Anatomy
- ☐ Genetics

INFECTIOUS DISEASES: REVISION CHECKLIST

Viral infections
- ☐ Hepatitis
- ☐ Infectious mononucleosis
- ☐ Chickenpox/measles/mumps
- ☐ AIDS/HIV
- ☐ Adenovirus
- ☐ Genital herpes
- ☐ Parvovirus
- ☐ Trypanosomiasis
- ☐ Leishmaniasis

Bacterial infections
- ☐ Venereal disease
- ☐ Brucellosis
- ☐ TB/BCG
- ☐ Tetanus
- ☐ Toxoplasmosis
- ☐ Typhoid/cholera
- ☐ *Bacteroides*
- ☐ *Haemophilus influenzae*
- ☐ *Helicobacter pylori*
- ☐ Lyme disease

- ☐ Meningitis
- ☐ Pneumonia
- ☐ *Staphylococcus*
- ☐ Diphtheria

- ☐ Tropical fever/splenomegaly
- ☐ Giardiasis
- ☐ *Pneumocystis carinii*
- ☐ Schistosomiasis

Routes of infection

- ☐ Transmission by insect bite
- ☐ Faecal–oral transmission

Tropical and protozoal infections

- ☐ Malaria

Miscellaneous

- ☐ *Chlamydia trachomatis*
- ☐ Other infections/diarrhoea
- ☐ Chronic infection and anaemia
- ☐ Infections and eosinophilia
- ☐ Prion disease

NEUROLOGY: REVISION CHECKLIST

Abnormalities of brain & cerebral circulation

- ☐ Dementia/Alzheimer's
- ☐ Transient ischaemic attacks
- ☐ Idiopathic intracranial hypertension/brain tumour
- ☐ Head injury
- ☐ Lateral medullary/circulatory syndromes
- ☐ Subdural haematoma
- ☐ Encephalitis
- ☐ Parietal lobe/frontal cortical lesions
- ☐ Temporal lobe epilepsy
- ☐ Amnesia
- ☐ Central pontine myelinolysis
- ☐ Cerebral abscess
- ☐ Creutzfeldt–Jakob disease
- ☐ EEG
- ☐ Intracranial calcification
- ☐ Midbrain (Parinaud) syndrome

- ☐ Normal pressure hydrocephalus
- ☐ Wernicke encephalopathy
- ☐ Subarachnoid haemorrhage

Spinal cord and peripheral nerve anatomy & lesions

- ☐ Innervation of specific muscles
- ☐ Median nerve/brachial plexus
- ☐ Posterior nerve root/spinal ganglia lesions
- ☐ Dorsal interosseous nerve
- ☐ Guillain–Barré
- ☐ Pyramidal tracts/posterior column pathways
- ☐ Sciatic nerve lesion
- ☐ Autonomic spondylosis
- ☐ Cervical spondylosis
- ☐ Motor neurone disease
- ☐ Paraesthesia
- ☐ Spinal cord lesions

☐ Polyneuropathy

Cranial nerve anatomy & lesions
☐ Facial nerve
☐ Cranial nerve lesions
☐ Third nerve palsy/pupillary reflex
☐ Bulbar palsy
☐ Internuclear ophthalmoplegia
☐ Fourth nerve palsy

Dyskinesias
☐ Ataxia
☐ Benign essential tremor
☐ Dyskinesia
☐ Parkinson disease
☐ Parkinson-Plus syndromes

Muscular disorders
☐ Duchenne muscular dystrophy
☐ Myotonic dystrophy
☐ Myaesthenia gravis

Miscellaneous
☐ Multiple sclerosis
☐ Headache/migraine
☐ Lumbar puncture/CSF
☐ Nystagmus
☐ Pseudofits
☐ Vertigo/dysarthria
☐ CNS involvement in AIDS
☐ Eye disorders

PSYCHIATRY: REVISION CHECKLIST

Psychotic disorders
☐ Schizophrenia
☐ Depression
☐ Mania
☐ Hallulcinations/delusions

Anxiety states/compulsive disorders
☐ Neurosis/psychogenic/conversion disorders
☐ Obsessional/compulsive disorders
☐ Panic attack

Eating disorders
☐ Anorexia nervosa
☐ Bulimia

Other cognitive disorders
☐ Differentiation of dementia and depression
☐ Acute confusional state

Miscellaneous
☐ Psychiatric manifestations of organic disease
☐ Alcohol dependency
☐ Insomnia
☐ Narcolepsy
☐ Endocrine causes of psychiatric disease
☐ Psychiatric manifestations in adolescence

INDEX

Locators refer to question number.

BASIC SCIENCES

INFECTIOUS DISEASES

NEUROLOGY

PSYCHIATRY